FOOD
for
FUEL

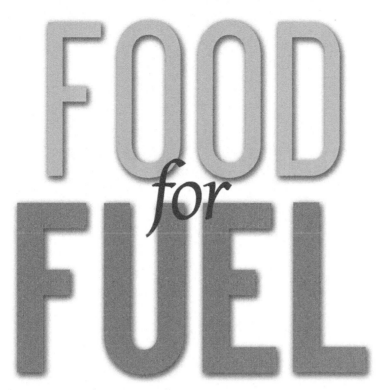

FOOD *for* FUEL

EAT LIKE A **BIRD** & LIVE LIKE A **KING** (OR **QUEEN**)!

M. Stephen Deneen

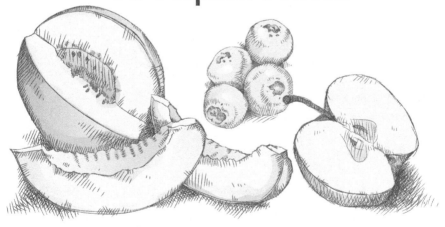

BLUE BUNGALOW BOOKS

©2016 by M. Stephen Deneen.
Published by Blue Bungalow Books.

ISBN: 978-152113-0636

Cover design by Paula Goldstein, www.bluebungalowdesign.com

To my loving wife Paula,
without whom there would be no book possible.
Thank you for your generous time, design chops, and love.

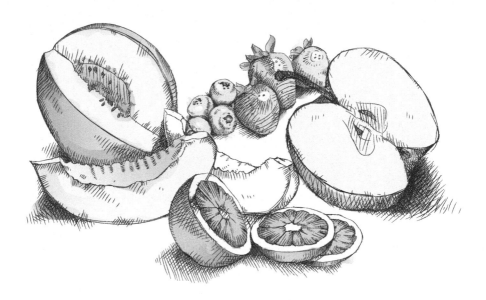

CONTENTS

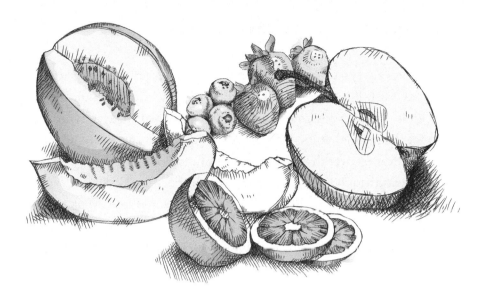

PREFACE

I began this project of writing a book on nutrition from an unusual perspective. I did not spend my career in medicine, nutrition or food science, but rather in the field of engineering.

After retirement I volunteered for years at an adult day care center, where we provided day services in nursing, socialization, and physical therapy for a large class of under served seniors. I quickly observed (and here my engineering talent was useful) that those seniors who had the most complicated health problems, were also those who were the most overweight, or obese.

There appeared to be an obvious correlation between obesity, and the most common combined conditions of heart disease, diabetes, and arthritis—the Big Three. This group had the most physical difficulty, especially with mobility. In my estimation, their obesity was dragging down their quality of life as compared to the minority group who had a more normal weight range.

I was always a slight kid. Even through college I maintained a size 30 waist. But, once I got into the working world, and building an adult life, I quickly gained weight that stubbornly stayed with me for the next 40 years. I stayed about 30 pounds overweight, and could never recover that 30-inch waist of my youth.

It wasn't for a lack of trying. I tried all the popular diets of each era, and always had about the same results. I would lose 10 or 12 pounds over six months, but then a year later I was right back to where I started, and often a few pounds worse. Like most people, I chalked this up to a lack of "will power".

A couple years ago, I once more took careful note of how many seniors I saw who were suffering from their obesity, and I could see I was headed for the same fate of gaining a few pounds with each passing year. This time, instead of trying another diet that I knew would never work, I decided to approach this as an engineering problem: Learn the physics principles. Learn the dynamics. Observe the problem in detail, and then craft a solution. That's the standard engineering practice.

It was then that I experienced the epiphany that led to this book: Food was never intended as entertainment. It was intended to be fuel for a complex and intricate machine—the human body. Our distant ancestors, the hunters and gatherers, had a primal understanding about food. They were not assaulted by endless advertisements to eat junk food. They had no pre-processed food at their disposal. What they had access to was Nature's bounty, and nothing else. Even artists who attempt to recreate scenes of this ancient life seem to understand that they would not be obese when relying upon nature. Our works of art always depict these ancestors as trim, muscular, and fit. Good artistic intuition!

From this point of view, from this model of nature's intent and intelligent scheme of life forms, from the lowliest to the highest, a most obvious hypothesis evolved: If we can ignore the artificial constructs and propaganda of those who simply want to profit from our over-consumption, and choose instead to follow the intelligence built right into every cell in our bodies, we too could gain the body originally intended by Nature. We too could be trim and fit throughout our entire life. In short, food was meant for fuel, and not entertainment.

Although my inspiration for the book was seeing too many seniors and retirees handicapped by obesity, people of any age will benefit by this knowledge. The younger you are when you recognize Nature, the better your entire life will be. *Food for Fuel,* is a lifetime commitment to good health, and not a passing fad.

M. Stephen Deneen

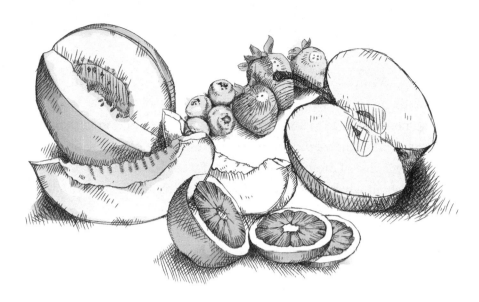

INTRODUCTION

Like millions of other Americans today I entered retirement considerably overweight and needing three different blood pressure medications. I knew I was overweight, but didn't realize I was just about to the standard of obesity. I told myself I could get rid of the extra pounds anytime I wanted, and often tried diets for a few months, but always without permanent success. My Body Mass Index (BMI) was 28 when it should be around 20. I had that all too typical "big belly" that is a feature of nearly all older men these days. In fact, I was not just overweight, I was a year or two from becoming obese.

Making things worse, my medication list was growing longer. Each year it seemed one new medication was being added. At the end of the year I was in the doctor's office for a regular consultation, and she said if my cholesterol worsened she would be adding a statin drug to my already long list of medications. A loud bell went off in my head. With New Year's just a week away, I took the opportunity, as we often do, to "start over" as a New Year's resolution. At the time, I had no idea where that would lead, or what the discoveries would soon be, but I knew I did not want to live the rest of my life on an ever longer list of drugs, to combat what was clearly an individual choice about what I was eating. My morning routine began with the pill box. This included:

* HCTZ for high blood pressure
* Atenolol for high blood pressure
* Lisinopril for high blood pressure
* Omeprazole for acid reflux disease (GERD)
* Prednisone for Polymyalgia Rheumatica (PMR)
* Metformin for a slight case of diabetes brought about as a side effect of Prednisone

And to this list, my doctor was about to add a statin drug? Enough was enough. I knew that the future was running downhill unless I took immediate control of my diet. Although I was over-weight, I was nowhere near the tragic overweight condition of so many of the other seniors I saw in the category of "morbid obesity." That term defines people that are 100 pounds or more overweight, or have a Body Mass Index (BMI) of 40 or more. It was no longer rare to see people in this condition everywhere I went. People too heavy to walk properly, were ending up in electric wheel chairs. Many with bad knees, but not able to get available knee replace-ments because doctors will not agree to operate on people whose weight is going to cause the replacement to fail. And yet, in the midst of all this pain and suffering, eating was still a thing to look forward to; a celebration of fun, entertainment, and socializing. Sure, diets were constantly discussed, but a quick look around would tell anyone that diets weren't working. Something went very wrong in modern western civilization, and it was on display everywhere I went. Long lists of medications were keeping very unhealthy individuals alive, but not living a healthy life.

This book is about nothing less than your personal revolution against the food industry. It is your way out of the worst trap in modern life—the food culture trap. In the months that followed my wake up call in the doctor's office, I discovered some painful truths, and at the same time a foolproof method for anyone to break this modern curse, and become the healthy person they once were in their youth.

Yes, no matter where you are today, no matter how overweight, no matter how many medications you are on, you can reverse all of that. You can regain your health, eliminate many medications, and it won't cost you a dime. There is no 12-step program to join, no special food to buy from the weight loss industry, no expensive supplements to buy from those TV infomercials promising you will lose weight. There are no gimmicks here of any kind—only very simple nutritional science that anyone can apply. The only requirement is that you can read, comprehend simple science, and have some willingness to regain your health and your life.

What I am going to present to you is what every primary care physician should be teaching their patients—but are not. It's what every school program should be teaching children—but are not. In fact, you will not find this information readily available in a concise way anywhere but in this simple book. No, I have not invented anything. What I have done is employ the scientific method to observe, measure, test, and then deduce the solution to permanent weight loss and better health. The result is this easy to understand book.

How do I know this works? I lost 35 pounds in 4 months, and got my BMI down to about 22 —so far. I have eliminated a blood pressure medication, medication for GERD, and my diabetes medication. I have more energy, more mobility, more alertness than I have had in 30 years. And, I am only half way through my journey. With a little more time, I expect to eliminate all the blood pressure medications. My diabetes has been cured. My GERD has been cured. My goal is to be medication free by the time one year has passed. According to my doctor, that will be possible if I get my BMI down to 20. You can do the same thing I did, and everything you need is right here in this short book.

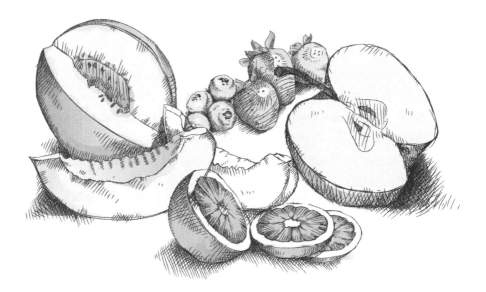

CHAPTER 1

Living in the *Food Culture*

Throughout this book I will use the term "food culture" to describe the way food has been transformed from nutrition to nonsense by the food manufacturing industry that surrounds us on all sides. How food became a source of our entertainment and pleasure at the direct expense of our health. How the food industry built a non-stop consumption machine for the purpose of generating ever increasing profits by ignoring the nutritional purpose of food—and even worse—by making us sick and disabled.

It begins from the moment you wake up in the morning. Turn on any of the popular morning TV shows and there will be a food segment, a celebrity chef, a new holiday recipe, or a new cookbook being pitched. It's new, delicious, entertaining and fun, you will be told. Your morning newspaper will be jam-packed with food advertisements and special deals. Everywhere you go during the day you will be surrounded by food opportunities: convenience stores, gas stations, fast food restaurants, vending carts, and mobile food trucks to follow the lunch crowds. Just keep your eyes open and consciously observe for a day or two. Every time you see any reference to food, just say the word "food" out loud to acknowledge it. In just a day or two you will have a new appreciation of how you are surrounded, day in and day out, by the allure of food.

If you go to events or entertainment venues you will quickly notice that even there you will be surrounded by food. Baseball parks are all about the food. Shopping malls have huge built-in food courts. Even the museums have attached fancy cafes to their operations. Your Facebook feed will be a constant stream of food videos, recipes, and pictures of food from your friends (even more than the cat videos). There is really nowhere you can go to escape food temptations.

At the grocery store, the number of manufactured food items grows every time you visit. If there was one flavor of a new snack food today, tomorrow there will be six new flavors of that item. The aisles dedicated to pure junk food are the largest and most plentiful aisles. Go ahead and see if you can even count the number of different potato chip offerings. The number and varieties of crackers, cookies, and high calorie snacks grows every year. The check out counter will be jammed with tabloids and magazines hawking new diets right alongside the food magazines hawking the newest recipes. "Eat more today!" "Start a new exciting diet today!" These two messages are the yin and yang of the food culture. You will always see them together, not just at the magazine racks, but on TV as well. They go hand-in-hand as the basic premise of the food industry. That industry makes money on both sides. They make money getting you overweight, and then they make money helping you try to lose weight. The weight loss industry is just another arm of the food industry. They want to sell you food too, but just a different kind of food. More about that later.

The expectation at home will be that you prepare three meals every day, and your family will expect lots of variety. You will be immersed in a relationship with food from morning till night. If you pay attention to it for a few days, you will see that food dominates your mental thought process. Buying, making, and consuming food is a day long attention demanding process. Of all the ideas and concepts and desires on our mind daily, food is the one demanding and getting the most attention. No wonder. We are stimulated about food non-stop by the advertising and media arms of the food industry. Where do you think all those recipes on Facebook come from?

That all immersive, constant, ever-present, ever-tempting food experience that invades our minds is what I call the food culture.

Once you are roped into it, you become their prisoner. It is not simply an accident or coincidence. Food is a major industry, and consuming food creates great wealth. Therefore, perpetually consuming more food, is the not so hidden agenda of thousands of food companies. Consuming food has been transformed from a biological concept into entertainment, sport, connoiseurship, status, and social currency. The idea of food as just nutrition has been totally lost. This onslaught of non-stop food advertising and promotion is fueled by the intentional psychological propaganda techniques invented in the 1920s by the father of Public Relations, Edward Bernays. Bernays showed industry how the minds of the masses can be made to adopt almost any position if the propaganda is directed with the right cues. He almost single-handedly created the consumer culture through the development of advanced propaganda techniques used in advertising.

Nutrition is at most a small advertising hook. At best, the advertisers attach words like "natural" or "organic" to food products as a small nod to nutrition. And at worst, nutrition is completely undermined by the push to consume more and more high profit snacks and junk foods. These ultra-processed foods now account for a whopping 57% of all calories consumed by Americans.

This immersion in the food culture has three very negative effects on the population. First is the obvious one—we are becoming obese at an alarming rate. And, that includes all age groups from young kids to seniors. The entire population is a valuable target for higher food consumption. The second effect is the rise in related health care costs. It begins with high blood pressure and high cholesterol, and continues right on up to diabetes, clogged arteries, bypass surgery, and in the extreme, organ transplants. There is no dispute that a significant part of our ever rising health care cost is directly related to obesity. There is plenty of dispute as to what can be done about this epidemic. The third major effect is the deterioration of our quality of life. Life is simply harder for the sick and obese. And when you add old age, the complications can make life miserable. We have the medical know-how to keep everyone alive and well into their 80s, even when they are in very bad health. A dozen pills a day will do it.

In addition to observing how food surrounds you, also observe the population, especially seniors. When you are in the grocery store, look carefully and count how many seniors you see that are thin, and walking upright without assistance. Compare that to how many you see that are overweight and bound to walkers, canes and electric shopping carts. I see a devastating ratio of about 1 to 3. It seems cruel to me what food is doing to our elderly population. It is ruining their golden years.

It's cavalier to announce, "They are doing it to themselves. It's their own fault." It's cavalier because human beings are not immune to propaganda and advertising. Even the best and most disciplined people can fall prey to a barrage of advertising. We can't look around and say that 3/4 of our population are weak, or incapable of good decision making. That would be absurd. They are where they are because that's what the food industry does to people in order to make ever increasing profits. Yes, we can assign some blame to individual weakness, but not all of it.

In 2016 we don't need to present a lot of evidence about obesity. The studies have been done, the analysis is complete, and there is no controversy. Our waistlines are growing steadily, and here are the basic statistics:

* 68% of adults are overweight, and 34% are obese.
* 32% of children are overweight, and 17% are obese.
* 30% of low income preschoolers are overweight or obese.

That is a shocking set of statistics. But, we don't need to rely on the statistics. A trip to the mall, the ballgame, or the above mentioned grocery store, will give you all the information you need to understand how dramatic this change has become in our society.

We can't fix this for everyone. We can't even think of changing the food culture as a whole. All we can think about here, is how to individually remove ourselves from the devastation and create our very own personal narrative about food, nutrition and health. That is the only path available to each of us as individuals.

This might be a good place to ask, "Does it make any difference if we are all obese? Aren't we all getting by just fine? Most of us are living well into our 80s. Doesn't that mean we're healthy?" Yes, it makes a difference. Try getting around at age 75 when you are 100 pounds or more overweight, your knees are both bone grinding on bone, you can't tie your own shoes laces, you can't go 15 minutes without visiting a bathroom to urinate from all the blood pressure medications, and you are constipated for days at a time.

Does that sound inviting? Well if you gain 5 pounds a year, which is very typical for many overweight people, that's what your future may look like. If you are still in your 40s or 50s, this is the time for preventative measures so that you never face that future. If you are already a senior, it's not to late to reverse most or all of the damage that has already been done.

You can avoid all of those problems caused by obesity if you get started today. You can move into your retired years as a thin, healthy person, needing no medications. You can be in good form for walking, golf, playing with your grandchildren, travel, and spending those last years in retirement feeling energetic and vital. The future is not sealed yet. No matter what your condition today, you can make dramatic changes that will greatly improve your condition. It's never too late to start.

The food culture is the outward consequence of the basic food business process. All businesses must grow, all the time. GM wants to sell more cars, Boeing wants to sell more airliners, and Apple wants to sell more iPhones. Every business seeks to grow their sales and unit volume every year. If the Ajax sausage company sold 1 million pounds of sausage last year, they will need to sell 2 million pounds this year to meet their growth objectives, and keep Wall Street and their stockholders happy. Growth of sales is the number one driver of stock prices. Any CEO who can't grow the stock price will soon enough be out on the street looking for a new job. More sales usually means more advertising, more promotion, more sales outlets, more chances for the consumer to find and buy the product. The food manufacturer, whether it is chocolate cakes or canned beans, doesn't care how the sales grow, as long as they continue to grow: more consumption is the imperative. You are just as good a target for more consumption as anyone else on the planet. If you ate 50 boxes of cereal last year, they want you to eat 60 boxes this year. Advertisers are not doctors or nutritionists. They make no assumptions or calculations about the suitability of their products for any individual. The ethics of the food industry do not consider the effects of national obesity. No food producer will put a warning on the label that reads: "Don't eat this if you are already obese." For the food business all consumption is good consumption, no matter who is doing the consuming.

Because of the relentless advertising assault, we soon enough succumb to the idea that we can eat all we want with no consequence. Our resistance is just overwhelmed by the delicious images, the talk, the advertisements, and of course, the wonderful taste and satisfaction of the food itself. Who doesn't love the taste of fried chicken or ice cream? Your taste buds tell you "good," the advertisements and promotions tell you "good," and the rest is just breaking down your resistance until you put it in the grocery cart, take it home and consume it. That entire process involves no scientific nutritional calculations. We"re no longer putting each food purchase into a context of total nutrition. But you say, "I read the nutrition labels!" Yes, most of us do. We can glean some idea about the food we are about to consume, but is that label really useful for all of us? For example, can you properly visualize the standard serving size of ice cream or potato chips? Can you properly judge serving size for you, and each of the members of your family? And, if you can, do you serve it all up properly, in the right proportions to be certain that no one in the family is overeating? A rare person you are if you can answer yes to all that. And probably a thin one! Most of us guess vaguely at serving size, and then grossly violate it when serving it up in a meal. Are you going to really be happy with 12 potato chips or 1 cup of ice cream? The science of nutrition doesn't lie. Your weight is a mostly simple calculation of calories in and calories burned. If you eat more than you burn over time, you are going to gain weight, and it matters not one iota what kind of calories those were. Too many salad calories is just as bad for your weight as too many ice cream calories. With such a simple balance as calories burned subtracted from calories in, it becomes obvious that unless we have precise understanding and control of those two numbers, we are turning over our nutrition and future health to the advertisers and simple desires of our taste buds. That's the danger of being deep in the food culture— science loses out to advertising and promotion.

Eating out is even worse than eating in. It doesn't much matter if you are at a fast food burger joint, or a white table cloth fancy restaurant. It's almost a certainty you will be over fed. When I began my working career in 1969, I liked eating lunch at the Woolworth's lunch counter just a few doors down from my office. I loved the grilled cheese sandwich at Woolworth's. It tasted great, and it only cost $1.10. I would put $1.25 on the counter when done, and be happy until dinner time. That grilled cheese sandwich was made from two pieces of wheat bread with one slice of American cheese in the middle. It was served with a couple of pickle slivers, and that was lunch. Yes, you could order French fries, but that was a different menu item, not an option on the sandwich itself. The sandwich was about 325 calories including the pickle. Just right for an adult lunch. Fast forward 45 years to today. Woolworth's is long gone, but let's suppose we stop at a deli and order that same grilled cheese sandwich. It will come with at least a pound of cheese between the bread slices, and often have three slices of bread. It will be served with a mountain of French fries, or potato salad, and of course the pickle too. But this modern version of the classic grilled cheese sandwich will easily add up to over 600 calories or more if you eat the sides that come with it. Portions have increased dramatically for two business reasons. First, a bigger meal will always feel like a better deal. That is, more for your money. Second, bigger meals come with higher prices, that makes the average sale to each customer higher. If you can serve 125 people during the lunch hour, which would you prefer as a businessman? 125 sales tickets at $3 for a simple grilled cheese, or 125 tickets at $7 for a whopper of a cheese sandwich with a mountain of fries? Restaurant owners intuitively understand the idea of giving a lot more food for just a little more money. It's a well-proven concept in the restaurant business. And people love it, as our waistlines amply prove.

Before we leave this topic, we have to talk about the great American hamburger. Have you paid attention to the size of the burgers being advertised on the TV? They are so large that the ad agencies have made a purposeful gimmick out of showing especially attractive and thin young women trying to take a bite of these enormous, multi-bun, multi-patty, bulging with cheese, wrapped in bacon, dripping with sauce, "gut bombs" called a hamburger. Some are 5" or 6" high. These new mega-burgers are topping out at 1,000 calories. That's the burger alone without the fries, and without the sugary soft drinks. Lunch in this fast food world can run an amazing 1600 calories or more. The average male requires about 2,200 calories a day to retain a stable weight. After a 1600 calorie lunch, what kind of dinner and snacks will be added to this total later? What kind of breakfast began the day? This problem of excessive proportions is visible everywhere in the restaurant environment, and not just limited to fast food. Order a pastrami or submarine sandwich at a deli and you will find yourself eating almost a day's worth of calories for lunch.

Portion problems are everywhere. There are take out pizza offers that include cinnamon buns with the pizza, or other super high calorie add-ons, sometimes built into the crust. Pizza comes with a built in feature for excessive consumption - no one can leave a piece in the box! Pizza just begs to be consumed in its entirely by it's neatly divided appearance. Where one piece might make a fair dinner, two is probably over the portion limit, and three is definitely going to be way over the top. I've seen ads for breakfast plates that include stacks of pancakes dripping in butter and syrup, alongside bacon, eggs and toast. Many of these breakfast specials begin at 1200 calories, and that is before the diner adds more butter or jam to the toast, more syrup, a glass of orange juice, or adds ketchup to the fried potatoes. These are not legitimate meals for most of the population. While they might be appropriate for a hard laboring miner, lumberjack, or deep sea fisherman, this is just a huge over indulgence for the rest of us who lead more sedentary lives.

Advertisers and restaurant chains are redefining for you what is a common sense portion. Not by any technical, scientific, or nutritional means, but simply by creating the images that dominate our daily lives. The TV commercials advertising these super-sized meals does not show them being eaten by morbidly obese people with insulin pumps and quadruple bypasses. They show them being consumed by happy, laughing, young, thin people. That is how new norms are created in the culture. The advertisers have no obligation to take our health under advisement. The only obligation that is certain is the obligation to help their clients grow the value of their stock. If you want, you can draw a direct correlation between our waistline and the stock price of food industry giants. This may seem a harsh moral judgment, but it is reality. Your waistline is considered fair game for all food related businesses, because the only principles that come under public scrutiny are economic ones. To some this may seem obvious, but it must be explained clearly and explicitly to understand the meaning of food culture. When we become active participants in this food culture, we are accepting and endorsing all these principles, that exclude any responsibility for our health.

I like the following analogy. When you enter an amusement park, you know intuitively there is some risk of injury involved in these high speed thrill rides. But you make the willing exchange of a small risk of danger for a lot of fun. You will accept the small risk of an accident in order to have a large likelihood of an afternoon of fun. This is a similar exchange you make when you enter the food culture.

You want the fun and the entertainment of all the delicious food, and you know there is an underlying risk to your health. But here's the difference: unlike the small risk of injury at the amusement park, the risk of entering the food culture is not small, it is immense, and it is almost always immediate. It's a very bad bargain for all of us. It's a risk we take multiple times a day for our entire life.

When you enter the food culture, there is no one there to protect you. No one is going to check to be sure that you have that safety belt locked around you before the ride takes off. No one is charged with actually monitoring your safety. You will not run into a waitperson who is going to ask, "Are you sure this is a good choice for you, considering your high cholesterol?" "You look overweight."

Did you know this breakfast has 1500 calories? You won't see a sign that says, "You must be this thin to order this super burger." Your doctor won't demand that you present them with a list of your meal choices. The FDA, or the government, is not standing by to bail you out of a pizza disaster. You are on your own, and being propelled forward by the world's greatest advertising minds. Minds who have spent their career redefining for you what is fun, what is normal, what is good, and what is valuable. How do you think you will stand up individually against an army of the world's greatest advertisers and brand managers?

When the food industry is asked about this unfair alignment against the consumer, they always have the same answer: "The consumer has a choice. All we do is provide that choice." That's the answer that excuses all excess and forgives all sins by advertisers— you had a choice. If you made the wrong one, they are not to blame. Everyone has heard this. Everyone has been trained to believe it. It's the corporate mantra in America. Well yes, you had a choice in a certain sense, but that choice is rigged heavily for you to make the wrong one. Sure, it's possible you could beat LeBron James in a game of one-on-one basketball, but really, how likely is it? My goal here is not to just place blame on the food providers, because they don't care, and that won't help you.

My goal is to provide you with the best defense possible against them. To up-armor you, and make it possible for you to get the upper hand against the impossibly well funded enemy. I want you to win physically, not just morally by placing blame. If they have the best creative brains in the country behind their advertising weapons, I will provide you with the bulletproof vest to make it through that war zone for your waistline. They will do what they will do, and I will show you how to defeat them. Your future is at risk, and you need a better system of self-defense.

Another important part of the food culture is the aggrandizement of food provided by the gourmets and "foodies" (slang term for those who love, admire and respect food of all kinds as a hobby). The gourmets are involved deeply with the preparation of exotic recipes and meals that express the talents and capabilities of the chef. The gourmets, foodies and epicureans are so involved in eating for pleasure that they represent the opposite pole from where we want to be in a program of eating for better health. We call it *food for fuel*. We can say that where the gourmets are living to eat, we want to eat to live.

Both foodies and epicureans are highly involved in creating the food culture directly. They are the cheerleaders, the recipe makers, the book authors, the TV show creators and hosts, and the promoters of new chefs and new restaurants. Their love of food also involves another disaster—the consumption of too much alcohol. Usually regarding wine, but often other spirits and beer as well. There may not be anything as contradictory to good health as excessive alcohol consumption. The need to avoid alcohol is not a matter of sin, or prudishness, it is a simple matter of avoiding toxins that further attack your health.

For foodies and gourmets every new food idea is an opportunity for excitement, fun and entertainment. Their houses are chock full of cookbooks and recipes. They will be found watching reality TV shows like, cooking competitions, celebrity chef challenges, and world travel that involves tasting local delicacies. Their purpose is clear— present food as a way to enhance their enjoyment through the senses. They may say their food is healthy and well balanced nutritionally, but not too many of these people are on the low end of the BMI scale. All you have to do is take a quick look at the physiques of the super star chefs of reality TV to see the end result of many years of this kind of cooking and eating. Are any of them really thin? We believe Epicureanism is incompatible with our program of *food for fuel*.

What the epicureans and foodies do properly acknowledge is that our manufactured foods, things found in boxes, cans and bags in the central aisles of the grocery store, are loaded with undesirable ingredients. These ingredients are present to enhance profitability for the maker, and not the health of the consumer. Preservatives for example, have the namesake job of making the packaged food last longer on the shelf. Often, three or more preservatives are used, and none of them has any positive nutritional benefit. Other artificial ingredients are there to create or enhance flavor, add color and create desirable texture. Those would be the ingredients with the extra long names you can't pronounce. Those are technically not foods, they are just chemical additives. As time goes on, the manufacturers and their food technicians become ever more clever at adding very low cost chemicals to the basic food stocks in order to create very high profit packaged products. This is particularly true with snack and junk food categories.

The larger danger of such manufactured and packaged food is their sugar, salt, and fat content. It didn't take long once food became industrialized for the makers to understand the preferred human taste and satisfaction profile. We humans are pretty simple to figure out. If a food has sugar, salt, or fat— or better yet all three—it thrills the palette of nearly everyone. Carrots or ice cream, which will make you smile?

Sugar

We need to understand two categories of sugar. First is naturally occurring sugar. This is the sugar that is intrinsic to a plants like bananas, broccoli or apples. Yes, even green vegetables have small amounts of natural sugars. Those are the sources of sugar we want to eat. "Added sugar" is simply sugar that has been refined from some source like sugar cane, or corn, and then added to a prepared, packaged food like cereal. Sugar is added generously to breakfast cereals that otherwise would be quite bland, and not a whole lot of fun to eat. Kids consume the most cereal because of it's convenience and ease of preparation for busy families. So they were targeted first with cereals loaded with added sugar. The brands are named after popular cartoon characters so that they can make easy identification through TV advertising. The colorful and cute Kellogg "Froot Loops" parrot is an example of cereal branding aimed at children. That cereal is 48% sugar by weight! I don't mind saying right now that if this is in your pantry, run fast and throw it directly into the garbage. The earlier we develop a taste for sugar, the more we want and the harder it will be to eliminate it from our diet. Added sugar is never necessary for nutrition. The sugars found in nature's food are all the sugar your body needs.

Food manufacturers are very clever about sugar. It is not always identified on the nutrition label as "sugar". Here are some of the many names of added sugar: Sucrose, Maltose, Dextrose, Fructose, Glucose, Galactose, Lactose, high Fructose corn syrup, Oligofructose, Glucose solids, maple syrup, Turbinado, and so many more the list is almost endless. Anything ending in "-ose" is going to be some form of sugar. Manufacturers want to add as much sugar as they possibly can because more sugar generates more sales. This applies equally to many so-called natural or health foods too. Which is why we like the simple rule that if there are any ingredients you don't immediately understand, put it back on the shelf and move on. You do not need these ultra-processed foods for any reason in your life. Our sugar consumption is rising dramatically because sugar is being added to virtually every packaged food we consume. In 1820 we consumed about 20 pounds of sugar a year. In 2016 we are consuming over 130 pounds of sugar per year.

That's better than 1/3 of a pound per day! The sooner you rid yourself of these foods, the healthier you will be. Start now.

Salt

Next on the hit list is salt. Salt is an effective natural preservative. But, it also is a flavor enhancing mineral that boosts, or supercharges whatever existing flavors are in the food. Something that is normally bland, and perhaps even tasteless, is salted to make it pop with more intense flavor. Salt is also an essential ingredient for creating texture in breads and cheeses. Salt chemically alters the structure of animal proteins. For example without salt, sausage would be hard to hold together. It's no wonder that nearly every manufactured food contains a lot of salt.

Salt is comprised of sodium plus chlorine to make Sodium Chloride (NaCl). The human body must have sodium to exist. It is one of many naturally occurring minerals necessary for proper operation of the body. This natural sodium is contained in sufficient quantity in vegetables. For example: artichokes, sweet potatoes, radishes, celery, carrots, broccoli and bell peppers—all contain natural sodium. One cup of raw celery contains 96 milligrams of sodium. Just by eating vegetables, you will be getting all the sodium your body requires. Just as with sugar, you need no "added salt" to your diet. And yet, salt is added profusely to almost all manufactured and ultra-processed foods. Example: The recommended daily allowance for healthy people is 2300mg of salt per day. For those with certain medical conditions, the requirement is lowered to 1500mg/day. A very common can of manufactured soup could easily contain 900mg of added salt per serving!

Some of those effects of added salt are clearly beneficial to the taste and enjoyment of food. If that's all there was to it, it would be a miracle mineral. But, salt comes with a heavy price tag. Salt works on your kidneys to make your body hold on to more water. This extra stored water raises your blood pressure, and puts strain on your kidneys, arteries, heart, and brain. This is why everyone with high blood pressure is advised to cut back on salt consumption. But, if you are heavily into the food culture, and eating from the center aisles of the grocery store, cutting back on salt will be almost impossible. It is the quintessential ingredient of cheap manufactured food. Everything that is manufactured, processed and put in a box, bag or can is loaded with salt. Salt is the bottom line cheapest flavor enhancer possible, and can make poor quality food taste acceptable. Salt is a huge profit maker for the food industry. Just like sugar, "added salt" is never needed in a human diet, unless you have some rare disease. All the sodium your body needs for optimum health is found naturally in whole food. So, just like sugar, get it out of your diet, and out of your cupboards.

Fats

Now that we have removed added sugar and added salt from our life, the next of the big three additives in factory food comes from fat.

Fats and oils are a large part of making food more desirable. They impart a smooth, glossy texture to foods. They enhance the color of foods and they provide a means to hold flavors longer. When fats and oils coat the tongue, they carry with them the flavors they were initially married to, and extend the experience of taste. That is one of the most powerful effects of fats and oils in our diets. Think of how salad dressing works. The underlying greens in the salad have mostly mild tastes. By adding oils mixed with spices, eating salad becomes an entirely different kind of experience. One that is more like eating ice cream than eating vegetables. The texture of the meal is made creamy, and the spicy flavors linger on the tongue.

Heavenly, right? But all of this heavenly taste and texture comes with the price of high cholesterol and clogged arteries.

Fats and oils are dense in calories. By weight, fats contain twice the calories of carbohydrates. The consequence of this is that too much fat creates too many calories. And lets always be clear on the maxim that "calories are calories." Eat more calories than you burn off, and you will gain weight. It is not a contested equation.

Our bodies must have fats and oils to survive and thrive. Fats are essential. They are a crucial means of delivering such vitamins as K, D, A and E. But, all of those nutritionally necessary fats can be found in natural, unprocessed foods. Foods such as nuts, avocados, eggs, fish, and of course meat, and poultry. Later, we will discuss the amounts of such foods that are needed for optimal health. For now, it's sufficient to say, that you don't ever need "added fats" found in manufactured foods, and I"m sorry to say, that includes cheese.

Here is a quick review of the five basic fats found in our diet.

Saturated Fat

This comes from our red meat, poultry and dairy products. Saturated fat raises your total cholesterol levels, and raises the Low Density Lipoprotein (LDL) cholesterol. LDL is often referred to as the "bad cholesterol."

Trans Fat

This is mostly a manufactured product made through a process called hydrogenation. These are the most unhealthy fats. They raise the LDL, and the work to lower the healthy High Density Lipoprotein (HDL). The result is an increase in risk for cardio-vascular disease. Trans fats are another highly profitable ingredient in processed foods. Trans fats are cheap to make, and in deep fryers can be used over and over without breaking down. That lowers the cost to make donuts and French fries. This is one fat you want to avoid at all costs. The FDA has mandated that all trans fat be eliminated from the America food supply by 2018. That's how bad they are for your health. If you see "partially hydrogenated" anything on the label, just put it down.

Monounsaturated Fatty Acids

These are the healthier fats. They can even lower your cholesterol, and help control insulin levels and blood sugar. They are commonly found in olive oil, avocados, and almonds, cashews and pecans.

Polyunsaturated Fatty Acids

This type of fat is found naturally in plant-based foods and oils. Soybean oil, corn oil, sunflower oil along with salmon, mackerel, herring and trout are all sources of polyunsaturated fats. These fats are considered less harmful to the heart than saturated fats, but not as desirable as monounsaturated fats.

Omega-3 Fatty Acids

This is a special kind of polyunsaturated fat that "might" help prevent heart attacks and coronary artery disease. This fat is most generally found in fatty fish like salmon, tuna, trout, mackerel and herring. It can also be found in flax seed, canola, nuts and seeds.

The bottom line regarding fats (and oils) is to avoid adding them to your food. You will get enough of the desired fats naturally within the natural foods you are eating. At most, you want to limit your calories from fats to less than 10% of your daily total. In a 1500 calorie diet, that means less than 150 calories from fats. A tablespoon of olive oil is 120 calories. So, you can see that it doesn't take much to over do it with added fats and oils. The most common use of added fats and oils are in cooking. In cooking, fats and oils are crucial to such techniques as browning and frying. The use of oils for heating foods means they can be cooked internally without burning the outside to a crisp. This is because oils are very efficient at heat transfer. This is the reason we do not want to do a lot of that style of cooking. And certainly never use deep frying in oil.

The Olive Oil Myth

This is the time to talk about olive oil. For years it has been proposed that olive oil is actually a beneficial food that improves health by lowering LDL cholesterol. This is highly suspect, and there are many new studies that question this effect. Since olive oil is a processed food product, it is better to leave it off your list all together along with all the other added fats and oils. Get the fats you need from eating whole, natural, fresh food.

What About Cheese?

Cheese is a heavily processed food loaded with saturated fats and salt. It is also very dense in calories compared to other foods.

Cheese begins with three strikes against it: It is high in saturated fat; high in sodium; and calorie dense. This is a food that is totally unnecessary in our diet, and yet is one of the most popular and most beloved foods, right next to ice cream. This is a food that should be consumed in very small amounts, if you can't take it off your list entirely.

We've covered the three worst ingredients of manufactured foods - sugar, salt and fat. What makes the discussion sometimes confusing in the world of food and nutrition, is that we need all these nutrients to survive. But, the important point to take from this is that we don't need them *added* to our food, if we just eat naturally. The processed food industry is always trying to tell us they are providing essential nutrients in their packaged food. That's a half truth. Yes, we need sugar, salt and fat to live, But no, we don't need them added to our foods just for enhancing flavor and texture.

QUICK REVIEW

✳   The food culture is an all-encompassing industrial advertising and entertainment environment that promotes overeating fast food,
junk food, and ultra-processed food as a means
of excitement, adventure, entertainment and pleasure.

✳   The results the food culture has had on Americans is an
overweight society with obesity and weight related disease
rising dramatically in the past 100 years since processed
food took over our diets.

✳   The processed food industry is loading packaged and convenience foods with excessive amounts of sugar, salt, and fats
to make this food almost addictive.

✳   To be healthy, thin, and fit, all we need to do is eliminate all
processed foods in favor of simple natural, whole foods.

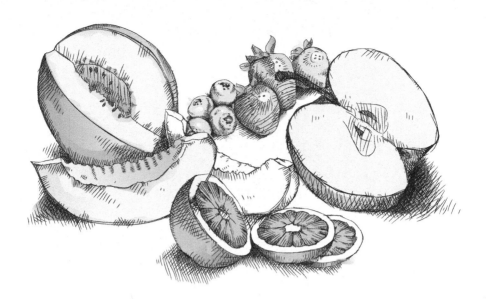

CHAPTER 2

Let's Talk About BMI

I am particularly sensitive to the problems of gaining weight with age. How many times have you heard seniors or retirees lamenting the good old days when they could wear that military uniform, or that wedding dress? For most people their early adult years represent their best fitness and lowest adult weight. Over the years, they get less exercise, eat just a little more each day, and eventually find themselves at some point in the overweight chart. How many of us still weigh what we did in college, or during our first job, or when we first joined the military? A few, yes. But, for most people those weights are a distant memory. People don't even consider that it would be possible to regain that position, but it is. You are not condemned to your current weight. I don't care how long you have been overweight, it's not a permanent setting that can't be changed. If you weighed 140 pounds as a 20 year old, and weigh 200 pounds

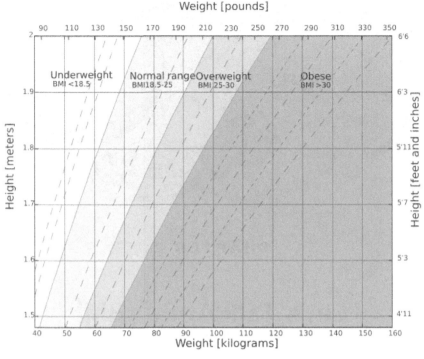

Body, Mass Index (BMI) chart.

today, you can get back to that 140 pounds. There is no physiological reason you can't. There are only practical reasons, having to do with your lifestyle, that prevent you from going back in time to a healthier weight.

Let's talk a little bit about BMI, "Body Mass Index", a means of having a convenient reference for our goal, and to measure our progress. People come in many sizes, shapes and bone structure. But no matter which kind of body you have, you don't want to carry excess body fat. The BMI measurement gives us a way to measure body fat by some simple calculations. It is well understood how much fat is needed for healthy operation. For men, it is about 15% of your body weight and for women a little higher, about 22%.

Those numbers represent the ideal conditions for a typical

adult. Those numbers might not be applicable to athletes, who may tone their body for higher performance by replacing some fat with more muscle, but this book is not about athletes, so I am going to focus only on average adult bodies. Knowing the typical body fat numbers for good health, we can do some standardized calculations and come up with a reference measure for BMI.

Let's see how the BMI chart works with an example named, Joe. Joe is 5' 7" and weighs 190 pounds. His current BMI of 30 is considered obese by all medical standards.

BMI Chart

Here is a typical BMI chart where all the computations have been made for you. You find your "height" in the vertical column on the right, and then follow to the left until you are under your "weight" at the top of the chart. For Joe, find his height of 5' 7" on the right-hand scale, then his weight of 190 pounds at the top. Where they meet is inside the dark orange "obese" area that represents a BMI greater than 30.

How much weight does Joe have to lose to get back into the normal yellow range? Normal is a BMI between 18.5 and 25. Again, start with his height of 5' 7" on the right-hand scale, and move left until you get into the yellow section. Yellow begins at about 155 pounds for Joe's height—a BMI of 25. That means Joe has to lose (190-155 = 35) 35 pounds to get back to a normal body weight.

Keep moving to the left to the end of the yellow section at about 120 pounds—BMI of 18.5. Joe's normal weight then, should be between 120 and 155 pounds to be in the normal BMI range. Joe has to lose (190-120 = 70) 70 pounds to get to the ideal, low end of the normal BMI scale.

Now, find your normal range. Begin with your height on the right-hand scale, and move all the way to the left until you enter the yellow area. Read the weight at the top. That's your maximum normal weight. Keep moving to the left to the end of the yellow area.

That's your minimum normal weight. How much do you have to lose to get into the high end of the normal BMI range? Move left to the end of the yellow range. How much do you have to lose to get the low end of the normal BMI scale? That is our goal!

The BMI chart provides a lot of latitude for "normal" weight. In Joe's case any weight from 120 pounds to 155 pounds would be considered normal. But if we are making a significant change to achieve the best health, my advice is to always aim for a BMI of 20, the lower part of the range. Throughout the rest of the book we will refer to a BMI of 20 as "fit and thin". There are many advantages to being fit and thin. There is much less stress on your aging knee and hip joints. And, if joints are already damaged, your doctor will have fewer reservations about performing replacement surgery. When you are thin, your risk of clogged arteries, high blood pressure and diabetes is greatly reduced. Those are the most common diseases in old age. If you are still young you have the opportunity to prevent those diseases from ever taking hold of you.

Being thin makes you more agile, and any exercise you choose to do is easier and puts less strain on your joints. You have more stamina, more energy, and less pain. Thin people are less likely to develop debilitating back problems. There is no health related down-side to attaining a BMI of 20.

Can you do that? Of course you can. Anyone can do it. It doesn't require preposterous ideas like will power, positive thinking or hypnosis. Nor will you need any special pills or other popular dieting tricks. It's a social and cultural shortfall that more doctors are not insisting their patients adopt this goal, and help them achieve it. For the most part, doctors have thrown their hands up in frustration about their patient's nutrition. They will often suggest patients' lose weight, but they rarely have a detailed plan or monitoring system that will help them achieve that goal. Primary care physicians should be putting every patient on this food as fuel plan. This is the road to optimal weight and optimal health. Let's keep going down the path.

QUICK REVIEW

* The simplest way to mark our progress toward ideal weight and optimal health is the Body Mass Index chart, or BMI calculator.
* The ideal range of BMI is 18.5 to 25. That defines a body fat content of 15% for men and around 22% for women.
* Anyone can change their diet and lifestyle to achieve a BMI of 20.

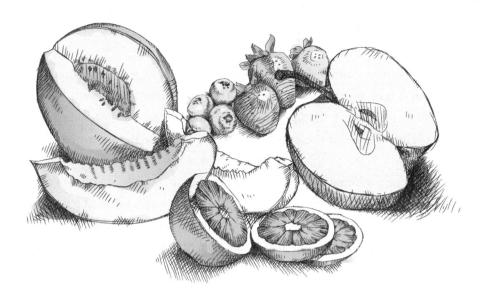

CHAPTER 3

Why Diets Don't Work

Every adult that has ever been overweight has tried a diet. Many have tried a dozen or more fad diets in their lifetimes. It's important to understand at the outset that this book is not a diet, it is a permanent change in your relationship to food. We are rejecting the food culture with all its ultra-processed foods, and accepting that the right relationship to food is to use *food as fuel*. Let's look at how this differs from a diet.

First of all, when people on are on a diet, they say "I'm on a diet, and can't eat that". They are defining a temporary condition.

They are on a diet now, and that means they will eventually be off the diet in the future. You can determine just from their comments that any diet they are on is going to be temporary. And, when they lose the number of pounds they had in mind for a weight loss goal, they will end the diet, and go back to whatever they were eating before the diet.

The dieter views the diet as a temporary change in condition because they are deeply involved in the food culture and eventually want to get back to that culture where food is entertaining and exciting. They are under the impression that if they use the temporary diet to lose some weight, they will be able to go back to the food culture and maintain this new weight. Of course, they are almost always wrong. It won't be long before they have regained all the weight they lost while on the diet, and very often added even more weight. At that point another diet is in order, and off they go bouncing back and forth between diets and the overeating food culture.

Researchers at UCLA* did an exhaustive analysis of 31 previous diet studies. Here's what they found:

> "You can initially lose 5 to 10 percent of your weight on any number of diets, but then the weight comes back." said Traci Mann, UCLA associate professor of psychology and lead author of the study. "We found that the majority of people regained all the weight, plus more. Sustained weight loss was found only in a small minority of participants, while complete weight regain was found in the majority. Diets do not lead to sustained weight loss or health benefits for the majority of people."

Mann and her co-authors conducted the most comprehensive and rigorous analysis of diet studies, analyzing 31 long-term studies.

"What happens to people on diets in the long run?" Mann asked. "Would they have been better off to not go on a diet at all? We decided to dig up and analyze every study that followed people on diets for two to five years. **We concluded most of them would have been better off not going on the diet at all.** Their weight would be pretty much the same, and their bodies would not suffer the wear and tear from losing weight and gaining it all back."

It is worth reading again! **Diets do not lead to sustained weight loss or health benefits for the majority of people.** Diets

*Source: http://newsroom.ucla.edu/releases/Dieting-Does-Not-Work- UCLA-Researchers-7832 April 3, 2007.

are fundamentally all the same. They involve variations of three basic tactics that are always doomed for long term failure.

* Will power
* Food substitution
* Short term duration

Will Power

Every diet requires the dieter to exercise will power in some degree or another. You want the chocolate cake, but using your will power you will deny yourself the cake and choose carrots instead. You want your baked potato to be stuffed with butter, cream and bacon bits, but using your will power you will settle for plain potato while you are on the diet. Most diet plans are filled with discussions about how you can increase your will power to be successful. They will paint wonderful pictures of your future to entice you to exercise more will power. Most of the promises and enticements involve dreams of improved sex, better relationships, and other fabulous outcomes, that will be yours if only you exercise a little more will power.

Will power, like physical ability, varies by person. Some have a lot, some have none at all. But to be sure, no one has infinite will power. A person can only resist constant temptations for so long, before giving in. Some diets actually go so far as to provide support groups, hot lines, or other means of bolstering your will power. Will power is needed to get you to do what you don't want to do. Using will power is an ongoing fight within yourself. Does that really sound like a strategy for success? Is your life going to boil down to fighting yourself internally every day? For how long? Does that sound healthful? What you gain by losing a little weight through will power will be offset by mental anguish. How can you possibly be asked to perpetually deny what you want, and continue to fail at doing it? Will power is not a useful strategy for regaining your health.

Substitution

The second strategy of diets is substitution. The diet industry wants you to substitute their special diet foods for the normal foods you have been overeating. Diet food,ugh! The mere mention of it brings a grimace to most people in the food culture. Diet food is not satisfying, doesn't taste good and if prepared and packaged by the diet company, will be downright expensive. In spite of that, substitution is the basis of most commercial diets—those being offered by makers of special prepared foods. The idea is simply to substitute these prepared low calorie meals for what you would normally eat. In this way, *calorie restriction and portion control* is achieved. The problem lies in these substitute foods themselves. I call them "faux foods."

Faux food is highly processed manufactured food items that have the *name, appearance and flavor* of highly desirable food, but without all the calories. How is that possible? Low calorie and low fat cakes, cookies, brownies, and ice cream are made by food technicians juggling dozens of chemical ingredients, artificial flavors, and preservatives to manufacture an approximate taste and feel of the original. Here's the ingredient list for a popular brand of commercial diet brownies, a real life example:

> **The Fiber One 90-calorie Chocolate Fudge Brownie from General Mills.** The ingredient list is quoted here from the label: Wheat flour bleached, Sugar, Chicory root extract, Chocolate Flavored Chips (sugar, palm kernel oil, cocoa processed with alkali, soy lecithin, milk, salt, natural flavor), Vegetable Oil (canola, palm, palm kernel), Fructose, Cocoa Processed with Alkali, Sugarcane Fiber, Vegetable Glycerin, Water. Contains 2% or less of: Dried Egg Whites, Leavening (baking soda, sodium aluminum phosphate), Cocoa, Natural Flavor, Corn Starch, Salt, Soy Lecithin, Milk, Xanthan Gum, Locust Bean Gum. Contains Wheat, Egg, Soy Milk: May Contain Peanut, Walnut, and Macadamia ingredients.

Simplified, it is a gooey mass of bleached flour, sugar, and oil stuck together with chemicals. Now this is being pitched as the healthful alternative to what is already an unhealthy mix of sugars, oils and flour, the original fudge brownie. Frankly, you are better off to just eat the real one made by Grandma with sugar, cocoa, butter and bleached wheat flour. At least it won't have the preservatives and chemicals.

The FDA has approved all those ingredients for use in food, so who am I to say they are not good for you? What I ask you to do is employ your common sense and intuition. Suppose you were offered the choice between a fresh picked apple and one of these chemical factory brownies—what does your intuition tell you is best for your health?

Faux food works to lower your caloric intake by substituting chemicals for real ingredients, but it will never change your eating habits, or your relationship to food. You will forever be committed to the idea that brownies are good to eat, if only you can find the lowest calorie brownie. All you are doing with faux foods is exchanging some calories for chemicals. This will commit you to a lifetime of misunderstanding food, and it's role in your health.

Substituting faux food is also temporary. When you are done with your diet, you will want to go right back to the real deal, the real brownies, and real ice cream. That's why the weight will always come back. The diet has accomplished no fundamental changes in your relationship to food. It has simply fooled you for a time, and given you a fake, temporary solution to the problem of overeating. The object of the faux food manufacturers is to keep you firmly and deeply committed to the food culture. You're eating their brand of brownies! You're eating their brand of ice cream! They don't care whether you are buying the high fat, high sugar brownie, or the low fat, lower sugar chemical brownie, as long as you are buying brownies! The diets that sell lots of this faux food even proclaim loudly in their advertising, "You get to eat all the foods you love!" And that's the problem. The food you love is killing you. You are in love with the wrong food, and eating way too much of it.

Diets Are Short Term

Diets begin and diets end. You stay on them until you achieve some goal for weight loss, and then you go right back to all the same foods you always enjoyed as a part of the food culture. It's a temporary fix to a lifetime problem. It's a patch, a band-aid, a plug in the dike. It's something you don't want to be doing, but are willing to do to achieve some weight loss. Very few people consider the diet as a lifelong commitment. If they did, they wouldn't say, "I'm on a diet," they would simply say, "don't eat that." Diets end in one of two ways. Either the weight goal has been met, or the will power has been exhausted. It actually doesn't matter which way it ends, because when it ends, you begin gaining weight again. Nothing at all has been done to address why or how you are overeating. You are overweight because you are overeating. There is no other answer, barring some rare disease conditions, like thyroid disease. Let's leave the medical problems to the doctors. If you suspect you have thyroid disease, or some other systemic disease of any kind, see your doctor and begin treatments. If you don't have one of those rare diseases, *you are overweight from overeating bad foods.* Say it out loud. That's what has to change. Calories in minus calories out, equals excess calories. Excess calories over time equals excess weight. We must now begin to deal seriously with the overeating problem. A diet is not the answer. It was never the answer, and it never will be the answer. It doesn't deal with the problem of overeating. It only deals with the problem of temporarily *reducing the calories* of what you are already overeating.

Commercial diets, where they sell you the substitute food to eat, are all based on the unworkable strategy of *will power, substitution of faux food, and temporary condition* of a diet.

Famous Doctor Diets

What about the popular "doctor diets"? The doctor diets don't all rely on selling you replacement food, but they offer you a list of approved and unapproved foods to achieve certain health goals like lowering cholesterol, reducing heart disease risk, and of course losing weight. These diets are an improvement over the fad diet because they generally advise better food, but just less of it. Although the doctor diets are a nutritional improvement over the straight commercial or fad diet, they still require will power and substitution, and they are usually considered temporary: "As soon as my cholesterol is normal, I can go off this restrictive diet." Doctor diets are known for long lists of "do's and don'ts". Don't eat this, don't eat that, stay away from this, reduce all of that. Once more, you need tremendous will power to follow these diets faithfully. "I love bacon and eggs, but my doctor has said I can't eat them." How long is that going to work out? It lasts until your will power is exhausted, and that is never long enough.

Doctor diets don't change your relationship with food. They fail to recognize at all how the food culture keeps you involved in eating for pleasure, amusement and excitement. Even if their recommendations are superior to the commercial and fad diets, you will rarely be able to maintain these restrictive diets for long because the doctor diets don't fundamentally address the problem of overeating. Like their commercial diet cousins, they ignore all that, and focus on good old substitution and will power. How would a person ever meet the problem head on if the problem of overeating is never discussed as a part of the diet?

Miracle Diets

The last category of diet is the "miracle diet". Everyone has heard this pitch on TV: "Eat all the cake and ice cream you want and lose weight!" Just take these special "fat burning" supplement pills, and the weight will magically disappear. These are not diets at all. They are just outright scams and frauds whose only goal is the sale of worthless dietary supplements. At best, these are benign ingredients packaged into pills with a deceptive label. At worst, these might be dangerous stimulants designed to speed up your metabolism. The most counter productive aspect to these miracle diets is the promise you can, "eat all you want." No, you can't. If you are ever to lose weight, and become healthy again, the plan must include reductions in how much you are eating. You can not "eat all you want" and lose weight unless you plan on removing the weight later with a chain-saw. Run the other way when presented with these magic diets. *You don't need any supplements of any kind to lose weight.*

When you are done with this book you will not be on a diet. You will not be on any kind of temporary plan, you will not be eating faux foods loaded with unpronounceable chemicals. And, you will not need any special will power. You will be actively eliminating the two causes of being overweight: an *improper relationship with food, and overeating.*

QUICK REVIEW

* Diets do not work. This has been proven beyond any doubt by bona fide researchers.

* Diets depend on will power, faux food substitution and temporary status. After dieting, the majority of all dieters gain all the weight back, and then some.

* The reason we are overweight is that we overeat bad foods encouraged by the omnipresent food culture around us.

* The only way to permanently lose weight and regain our health is to reject the food culture and adopt a new relationship with food, *food for fuel.*

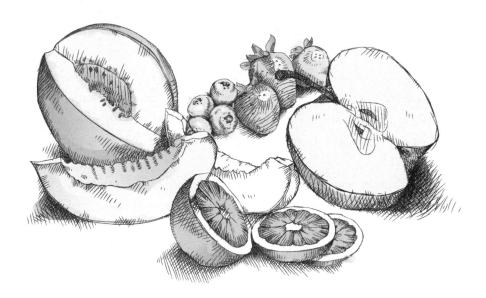

CHAPTER 4

Breaking Up with the Food Culture

Some relationships are just plain bad for us, and our relationship with food has become downright toxic. The only way out is to break up with the food culture. The romance with food is over. Your mind has been ruled by food, your body has been devastated by food, and now it is time to recover, renew, and start over with food in its proper and rightful place, *food as fuel*.

We were never biologically intended to have such a romantic, all-encompassing affair with food. Our love of ice cream, brownies and deep fried chicken has provided endless amusement, fun, excitement and entertainment, but now it is killing us. Are we going to allow this relationship to kill us, or are we going to take action and fix it? It is never too late to regain control of our eating habits and return to a healthy body. No matter your current weight you can recover, rebuild, and become thin, healthy and energetic again. The body has an amazing recovery capability, if only you give it a fighting chance. You do not need surgery, special drugs, pills, supplements or gurus to restore your body to optimal weight and good health. You only need the right information and a desire to permanently improve your health.

Food was never intended to be entertainment, or an amusement. Food was not intended to be an emotional support mechanism.

Food is not a substitute for love, sex or happiness. Food has only one biological purpose—to keep the body operating in peak health.

And for many thousands of years, that was the main role of food. It wasn't until food became a for-profit industry in the early 20th century that the purpose of food became grossly distorted to serve the goals of the industrial food manufacturers. The rise of mass advertising media, like magazines and television, allowed food producers to sell the public on consuming food for fun.

We're always careful to put the proper fuel in our cars, tractors and machines. We are careful to feed our pets the best nutrition possible. Mothers are careful to assure that their infants are properly fed. But when it comes to ourselves, we don't even eat as well as our dogs. With our own adult nutrition, we have thrown all caution to the wind. Nothing is off limits as long as it tastes good. It's as though we have lost all common sense when it comes to our own nutrition. We ignore warnings from science, government, family, friends and doctors alike. After many years of ignoring all the warnings we are stuck with an overweight or obese body and seemingly no way to get well. We are drowning in a sea of food culture advertising and surrounded on all sides by thousands of delicious tasting, oh so tempting garbage foods that fill the aisles of the grocery stores. How can we fight that overwhelming enemy of good health?

Science knows with almost perfect precision what the body

needs for optimum operation. But we allowed ourselves to be deceived and overwhelmed, accepting the ideas that food should amuse and entertain us. Now comes the celebrity chef with the exciting new recipes! Now comes the food magazines at the checkout counter tempting us with those gorgeous cover shots of decadent desserts! Now comes the reality cooking shows, cooking contests, fancy restaurants, fast food chains, and the massive grocery stores busting at the seams with junk food! It's no wonder we lost the battle. We've all been sucked into this vortex of food as adventure and fun. Now, we must retake the control of the reigns and exit the food culture for good. We must leave it all behind with one sharp turn putting it all in the rear view mirror for once and for all. That's how we break up with the food culture for good.

The food culture is a fantasy. It promises you will meet a sexy new partner, travel the world eating exotic foods, and have amazing life changing experiences just by eating a bag of potato chips, or an instant cream pie. It promises that if only you learn French cooking, or how to barbecue, you will meet and impress fascinating new friends. It promises that learning how to find fine wines and exotic micro-brews will bring new pleasure to your life. It promises you that the right BBQ and beer will bring more friends and sexy women to your man cave for Sunday football. That's the wonderful fantasy of the ubiquitous food culture. But you know by now none of those dreams came true, did they? You know in your heart that the only thing that ever happened was you got fat, and slow, and tired, and sick. You know in your heart that ice cream, deep fried chicken and potato chips never brought you a day of happiness. The food culture is one cruel hoax after another. Lies piled upon lies and deception. A total fraud.

The reality is being too overweight to walk, blown knee joints, a life of medication, diabetes monitoring, daily insulin shots, coronary bypass operations, and sitting around the house watching TV because you are too large to move around comfortably. Too large to fit in a car seat or an airplane seat. Too large for that beach bikini. Too large to go snorkeling or hiking, or sailing with all those new imaginary cool friends promised in the food commercials. So, let's admit we need a new strategy. Let's admit we must change.

How about another diet? The diet industry is just the flip side of the food culture coin. The diet industry keeps you tied firmly into the food culture with its faux foods, prepared chemical meals, and calorie counting systems that don't produce life long results. When the diet is over, and all diets come to an end, you will be as deep into the food culture as they day you began the diet. And you will be a little poorer. The weight you lost was nothing but the temporary exercise of will power. Since you haven't changed your relationship to food, you will be right back to square one and eating all the wrong foods.

"Breaking up is hard to do." Well, that's what Neil Sedaka said. Yes it is hard, but like any breakup it only has to happen once, and then you are over it. No, it doesn't take will power. If you think it takes will power, you need to re-read the previous chapters. Will power is the ability to resist your desires for a short period of time. When you really break off a relationship, what you are breaking off is the desire itself, not just the temporary ability to resist temptation. If it seems hard, or impossible, you may not be ready or convinced yet. Keep reading.

By breaking up with the food culture we are going to take sensible control of our internal biology, and begin to treat our bodies right. We are going to use the best available science and fully optimize our biological systems. Within just a few weeks you will feel a remarkable difference in health, vitality and energy. That's how fast the body can react to the proper nutrition. You will be losing weight without relying on will power. In a few months you will be eliminating medications because as your system improves, those common diseases caused by overeating will begin to fade into the distance. If you have high blood pressure, high cholesterol and diabetes, you may very well eliminate all those disease symptoms within a year. This will not be temporary, as it is in fad diets, but permanent. Your body replaces cells at the rate of 50 billion per day. Within a few months, you will have an entirely new body. One that is working for you, with you, instead of against you. Anyone can do this. Nothing special is needed, and it's absolutely free. There are pills to buy, no gimmicks required, no faux foods to make. No kidding! That's what breaking up with the food culture will do. It will radically change your life.

How exactly do we break up with the food culture? What do we even mean by all this? Let me begin with this quote: "Our own physical body possesses a wisdom that we who inhabit the body lack. We give it orders that make no sense."—Henry Miller

Our bodies have a built-in intelligence. Every one of our trillion cells knows exactly how to maintain itself, repair itself, replace itself. Those instructions are built into the DNA. We've been around for about 100,000 years in our current human form. We survived for 95,000 of those years without manufacturing contrived chemical foods like bread, deep fried chicken and chocolate cake. The human species survived on plants and animals found in nature. We have gradually complicated our diet by the use of manufactured fake foods. These unnatural foods multiplied, and eventually created an entire artificial world called the food culture. In this new world, eating became an adventure divorced entirely from the body's built-in intelligence. In place of nutrition, your body was being fed garbage that it had to fight off just to remain alive.

Breaking up means acknowledging what you already know. Seeing the toxic food industry as you have always known it is. It means finally putting our bodies ahead of their profits. It means growing into the real sensation of what a healthy body feels like. It means showing a little strength to tell the rest of the world you are no longer a sucker for the toxic food industry. It means seeing the right path, and taking it in spite of what others will think about you. It means being brave enough to be called "kooky" by your family and friends, who may remain stuck in the food culture their entire lives. It means accepting the universal and obvious truth that the built-in intelligence of every cell of our body is only seeking real fuel in order to perform at it's optimum level. Feed it garbage and you will be sick. Feed it fuel and you will be healthy. It means you stop following that food pied piper that is leading you from one fad to another. It means you stop giving your time and attention to food magazines, food TV shows, new restaurants, new recipes, food blogs, new cookbooks. It means you take all that time and energy you wasted on food culture, and use it for something creative, something new, something healthy and beneficial. It means you free yourself from keeping up with food fads, and fad diets.

The food industry will carry on fine without you. Others will find you peculiar. Your family and friends will argue with you. They will say you are being extreme, radical, and foolish. You are a revolutionary fighting the absurd governing body of food, and following a reformed, intelligent path to better health and happiness. And soon, you will be free of the unhealthy body that has weighed you down for years. Let's get started with some actions to take when breaking up with the food culture.

Step 1   Stop Cooking and Start Eating!

The idea of preparing elaborate meals from recipes using multiple ingredients and many spices is unnecessary, and it can be stopped immediately. Of course there are some simple soups and stir fries you can make, but they are primarily just a matter of blending and heating the few ingredients. You will be eating primarily "single ingredient foods", real foods, natural foods. They don't require spices, sauces, or heavy modifications through cooking techniques. Some of the vegetables can be steamed, and the very small portions of meat and poultry can be flame broiled or cooked on a BBQ. But those meals do not require any special ingredients.

Meals were never this simple and healthy. What to eat is coming up next. For now, ditch the cookbooks and recipe boxes. You don't need any of that. There is no need at all for fancy preparation. Eating the old way is the path to overeating the wrong foods. Many years of the old way is what got you into the unhealthy predicament that we want to now reverse.

Most old school recipes create the same problems as processed foods. They add too much of the three ingredients we don't want: sugar, salt and fat. This is especially true of baked goods like pies, cakes, cookies and pastries. Those are foods you never want to make, and should only eat on the rarest occasion. Once a year would be about right!

Old school cooking from exotic recipes focus exclusively on taste as the primary rationale. The object is to create memorable experience, comfort and satisfaction using food. But as we have learned, that's not the true natural purpose of food. We want the number one purpose to be health and nutrition with taste and comfort taking a strictly secondary role. This doesn't mean your meals will be tasteless. It means your meals will focus on natural flavors that you will soon enough be satisfied without using extraneous ingredients.

Step 2   Empty the Refrigerator!

Get rid of all the processed, chemical-laden foods immediately. These are usually in the form of dressings, spreads, cheeses and oils. If there is more than 3 ingredients on the label, dump it. You will no longer have a need for all these chemicals. Throw out anything that is made from wheat. Breads, pastas, rolls, cakes, muffins, pastries—

anything at all that contains wheat, wheat gluten or processed wheat grains. These highly processed, highly manufactured foods are not in your future. Throw out the frozen dinners, frozen waffles, pancakes, jams, jellies, and cheeses. If the meat is fresh, unprocessed, or minimally processed, keep it. Colas, beer, and anything artificially sweetened goes out. Fruit juice is OK, but avoid extra sweetened juices like cranberry, that is often loaded with high fructose corn syrup (HFC) in order to make a bitter fruit more palatable. Save fresh fruit and vegetables. Save frozen vegetables if they are not swimming in artificial and chemical sauces.

Step 3   Go Shopping!

Try to pick a grocery store with the best selection of fresh fruits and vegetables. Even better is any local farmers markets. In grocery stores, avoid all the center aisles where the manufactured packaged food is sold. Stay on the outside ring of the store where fresh food is sold. Select any of the fresh foods you already know you like. For starters, nothing is off the list. Choose what fresh foods you like and get plenty of it. This stuff is the core of your future meals. Select a good mix of vegetables, fruits, nuts and seeds. However, be sensitive to how much of the nuts and seeds you consume. A little goes a long way. Those are very high calorie dense foods. A few ounces a day would be more than enough. Buy fresh juices. Buy bags of frozen plain vegetables (no sauce). They are easy to prepare and keep for a long time. Explore—try some fruits and vegetables you have never eaten before. Experiment!

When you get to the butcher counter, select some small portions of pork, beef, fish or chicken. We need to add a few ounces of animal protein at least a few times per week. Lean beefsteak is expensive, but you will not be eating more than a few ounces at any given meal a few times a week. I like putting my beef into vegetable beef soup. You can also put lean chicken breast into chicken salad, or chicken soup. Buy quality. Since you are consuming much less meat, you can afford better, organic quality meats and poultry.

Step 4   Throw Out the Packaged Food in the Cupboards!

Most pantries and cabinets are filled with boxes and cans of manufactured industrial food. Macaroni and cheese, soups, casserole helper, potato chips, pretzels, crackers of all kind, cookies, pasta, cake mix, cornbread, baked beans . . . get rid of it all. You don't need anything in those boxes and cans. It has minimal real food value. It is loaded with sugar, salt, fat, and artificial chemicals.

There are a few exceptions. There are some dry soups, and even some canned soups, that are low in salt, sugar and fat. Also, beans that are not swimming in barbecue sauce. But keep in mind, all these prepared foods rely on added salt and spice to create intense flavors. These intense flavors are designed to keep you hooked on these manufactured foods. You want to get off of that habit.

The more you depend on these packaged foods, the longer it takes to adjust to the taste of fresh and natural foods. Your first judgment about whether to keep it or not should be based on the salt content. When you see 700mg of sodium per serving, get rid of it. If it is under 200mg per serving, it is edible. After salt, look for the number and kind of preservatives. If the list is long with complicated names get rid of it.

Step 5   Get Rid of the Bread and Pasta

Because modern *hybridized* wheat strains contains proteins that actually cause the hunger switch to turn ON, we want to stay totally clear of all products that contain wheat and wheat products. For wheat, there are no exceptions. Any wheat products you consume will create more hunger and promote overeating. Almost all wheat grown now in the USA is hybridized. These new wheat varieties have proteins that turn on the hunger switch in the brain. The more you eat, the more you will want to eat. Our reference is Dr. William Davis, author of **Wheat Belly Diet**. Although we don't believe in diets per se as a weight loss strategy, we do believe in doctor Davis' evidence that modern wheat is a contributing cause of obesity. Wheat is out! Breads and pasta are highly processed foods. We just don't need bread and pasta for good nutrition. And watch out for *wheat as an ingredient* in foods you would never guess needs wheat.

Wheat, in all it's forms, appears in numerous manufactured foods as an additive. Particularly wheat gluten. It is unnecessary for health in any way. It is a completely extraneous food product that only serves secondary purposes, not nutritional purposes. Breads and pastas are the cornerstone of the food culture. This is the time to leave that in the dustbin where it all belongs.

Eliminating wheat products will be one of the most controversial aspects of your new relationship with food. The USDA has been recommending whole grains as a major part of our diet since the inception of the food pyramid. What's important to remember about the USDA's role in our diets is that the USDA is an economic and political organization, not a health organization. The USDA is charged with helping to grow agribusiness in the United States. Their recommendations, like the food pyramid, represent that goal of advancing the largest segments of the agribusiness. We should never consult the USDA for our notions about nutrition. We will have no problem getting all the healthy foods we need without any wheat products.

Step 6   Get Rid of the Cookbooks!

Cookbooks are another cornerstone of the food culture. The cultural icons of cooking like, Martha Stewart, Julia Child, Bobby Flay, Mario Batali, and the Barefoot Contessa, make cooking and eating a culturally significant pastime, and badge of sophistication.

Cookbooks are the primary hook used to keep people chasing

the fantasy of a better life through the foolishness of using food as an amusement and source of pleasure. You may at first cry over the loss, but that's why I call this a breakup—it's not easy. You may even shed some tears.

You don't need any cookbooks. If you can boil water or heat a wok, you know enough about cooking to be healthy, vibrant, fit and thin. You do not need to cook! The body does not require fancy French cooking, Asian fusion cooking, Southern comfort cooking, or Grandma's German recipes to achieve optimum health. It needs only a little bit of some very simple natural foods. You can not make one iota of improvement in the *food for fuel* program by cooking foods according to fancy complicated recipes. Give all those cookbooks and recipe boxes to another fool, but don't give them to someone you love. Use the extra shelf space for good literature, that will actually help you out in life.

Remember tossing out all those photographs of your ex-spouse after the divorce? Yes, it's painful in one aspect, and yet liberating at the same time. It is a must-do for any good breakup. Cookbooks are the ultimate embrace of the food culture. You must exit completely. Doing so is why you won't need will power for this plan. If you hang on to all those cookbooks, you will be tempted to use them, and only will power will prevent you from back sliding. Why do that? Break up for real. Be bold enough, smart enough, to know what is right and what is wrong. Get the temptation out of your house. *Food is fuel*, not entertainment. But have no worries. After you shed all those excess pounds, you will look back and wonder why you hadn't done it sooner.

Step 7   Turn Off the Cooking Shows!

Cooking shows are the infomercials for the food culture. There are entire TV networks dedicated to the gods of the food culture. Turn it off forever. It doesn't matter what the celebrity chefs are cooking today. It doesn't matter who is wining the latest chef contest, or food shopping contest. Don't get sucked in to this world of cooking and food experimentation. There's nothing on that network about scientific nutrition. There might be shows on diets, but you don't need a diet for all the reasons we have explained. Diets are just the flip side of the food culture coin and have no real value to your long term health. Just like the cookbooks, this is a painful change that is a necessary part of the breakup. Rid yourself of the temptations of the food culture, by just turning off those cooking shows.

Step 8   Cancel Your Dinner Reservations!

There's nothing for you in fine dining restaurants except highly prepared foods with too many unhealthy ingredients. Restaurants are the temples of the food culture, and the chefs are the high priests. The restaurants are in charge of keeping you in the game, keeping you in the fantasy that excitement and adventure is the reason for food. These are the professionals that are showing you how it is done, and in the process giving you hope you can also do this at home. To make it worse, they will be overfeeding you with generally huge portions that are helping you to overeat. Part of breaking up is losing those old friends that helped you maintain the bad behaviors. If you had a drug addiction, you wouldn't want to be hanging out with drug users. It may sound impossible to enjoy life without restaurants, but it is not. There's plenty you can do with your new healthier body than going out to pay for the privilege of overeating. In the future, there may be restaurants that are offering natural, un-adulterated *food for fuel* meals. Right now, I don't know of any, so the best advice is to give them up, and save eating out for the truly rare occasions and celebrations that are unique. At most, a few times a year. And, when you do choose to dine at restaurants, don't be afraid to leave half your plate behind, and be sure to skip out on dessert.

There's your starting list of activities. Eight steps for breaking up with the food culture. Sure, it sounds like a lot, it sounds hard, and it represents a big change. But, consider for a moment that it's all you have to do in order to get your health back. There's nothing on that list that costs a dime aside from shopping for some new fresh food. There's no surgery, no pills, no bogus supplements to invest in. Really, can you think of a better bargain on this planet? Give your new revolutionary *food for fuel* program a try, and in a couple of weeks look back at all the people you know still stuck in the fantasy of the food culture. They will be overweight, over medicated, and underactive, while you will be starting to feel the new health and vigor takeover your own body. The difference will be so clear there will be no more looking back and second guessing.

QUICK REVIEW

*   The food culture offers nothing but empty promises of a life that leads to overeating and bad health.

*   Break up with the food culture and adopt a *food as fuel* nutritional view of food in place of the old school pleasure principle of food.

*   The eight simple steps for breaking up with the food culture will cost you nothing!

*   Save dining out for very special circumstances, and be sure to skip dessert.

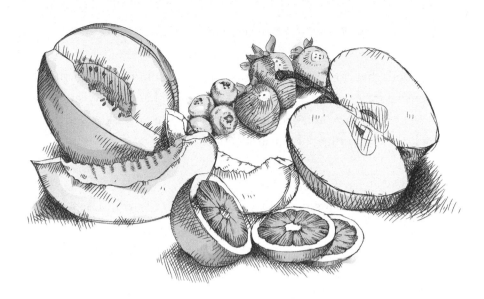

CHAPTER 5

Nature's Food and You

We've now come to the best part— what is it you are going to eat? How fortunate must we humans be that nature has provided all we need in very simple forms that are plentiful and easy to access? Speaking nutritionally, the food requirements for perfect health amount to *water, carbohydrates, proteins, fats and minerals.* We will not be going into classroom level detail on nutrition in this book, just explaining the basic essentials required for optimal health. We will skip nothing important, but we will simplify for brevity. I highly recommend *Nutrition for Dummies* by Carol Ann Rinzler, published by Wiley. It is available on Amazon.com if you want to have more scientific detail. What I am going to prove to you is that absolutely everything you need for optimal nutrition and excellent health, is contained in a few of the simplest foods on the planet, available at any grocery store. Foods that nature supplies in abundance.

Foods that do not require recipes, exotic cooking, foreign and expensive spices, or special preparation. Foods that actually suffer by over preparation and cooking. Mother Nature never knew about Chicken Cordon Blue, or Macaroni and Cheese!

Protein

Protein is the building block of all muscle and cells. All these foods are high in protein: poultry, seafood, cheese, milk, beans and peas, lentils, yogurt, eggs, soy, nuts, and seeds. Men and women need about 55 and 45 grams of protein a day respectively. Here are some simple examples of protein content.

* ✳ 3 ounces of meat has 21 grams
* ✳ 8 ounces of meat has over 50 grams
* ✳ 8 ounces of yogurt has 11 grams
* ✳ 8 ounces (one cup) has milk is 8 grams
* ✳ 8 ounces of dry beans has 11 grams

Special Note About Yogurt

In the old days, yogurt meant natural yogurt with nothing added to it. It's a bit bland and sour. It's not sweet. Today, there is an explosion of yogurt brands that take up a huge portion of the refrigerated aisle of the grocery store. Nearly all of these are just "sugar delivery systems." They are loaded with fruit, fruit syrup, High Fructose Corn Syrup, and other sweeteners to make sour yogurt into a dessert food, highly rich in calories. Whatever benefit yogurt may have is negated by all the sugar content. I don't recommend eating these on a regular basis. It's just about as bad as drinking soda pop, and in some cases worse. I would also never eat the artificially sweetened versions that amount to "chemical delivery systems." If you can eat plain strained yogurt (Greek-style sour yogurt) it is beneficial. If not, skip it.

Carbohydrates

Carbohydrates are your main source of energy. A carbohydrate is string of glucose molecules bonded together in a matrix. When we digest carbohydrates, we break the bonds and create individual glucose molecules in the small intestine. This glucose is carried by the blood stream to every cell in the body, where the glucose is burned directly as energy for the cells to complete their individual jobs. If you had no carbohydrates, the body would begin breaking down muscle for energy—a process we do not want to activate.

Carbohydrates come in two varieties: "simple carbohydrates" are made of sugar and fructose. They need little work by the digestive system before entering the blood stream as glucose. Better for us are the *complex carbohydrates*, that need more work and time to breakdown in the digestive system before being released as glucose. This provides more even energy throughout the day.

Complex carbs are found in beans, nuts and vegetables. On average we need about 130 grams of carbohydrates per day. But, because carbohydrates are the energy producer, you will need more if you are exercising a lot, and less if you are mostly sedentary.

Around half of your daily calories should be from carbohydrates. When people think of carbohydrates they immediately think of potatoes, breads, pasta, cereals and grains. But, we are eliminating wheat products, and therefore our carbohydrates are going to come from healthier sources like bananas, broccoli, pears, corn, potatoes, apples, leafy greens, sweet potatoes, rice, figs and berries.

To simplify this even further, just assume we are going to get all of our carbohydrates from fruits and vegetables. Get breads and grains out of your head as we previously explained. Our great cities and civilizations were built on the ideas behind growing, storing and processing grains. Today, we don't need to rely on storing food through winters and bad seasons because we have massive transportation systems that can move a fresh tomato thousands of miles in any direction within a few days. Fresh food is available year round nearly everywhere on earth. (Note: that is not to minimize the great political difficulties that some populations have in getting access to any food, of any kind, including grains and breads.) Because we have such access to fresh foods, natural foods, we can give up our reliance on old systems of eating stored grains. We are moving past mere survival, and taking advantage of our opportunity to thrive in the best possible health. It may seem heretical, but you do not need breads and pastas for carbohydrates.

Fats

It may sound illogical when we are trying to eliminate *excess fat* from our bodies, but our bodies also need certain nutritional fats to function. Science calls them "lipids," and the study of all the kinds of lipids is a text book unto itself. We do not need to study that hard here, and once more I refer you to a basic nutrition book if you need to know all the categories of fats, and how each operates. Fats are needed to build the cell wall. *We can not live without them.* But, the amount we need is relatively small, and can easily be obtained from some simple natural foods. Fats come in the following types. Be sure to note the differences.

Monounsaturated Fats

These are healthy fats and include oils like olive oil, canola oil, peanut oil, safflower oil and sesame oil along with nuts, seeds, avocado and peanut butter.

Polyunsaturated Fats

Walnuts, seeds, salmon, tuna, and non-GMO tofu are typical foods with healthy polyunsaturated fat. A special kind of polyunsaturated fat are the Omega-3 and Omega-6 essential fats. They are called essential because they body can not synthesize them from raw ingredients. They must be consumed in original form. The best foods for these essential fatty acids are: fish and shellfish, flaxseed (linseed) and flaxseed oil, hemp seed, olive oil, soya oil, canola (rapeseed) oil, chia seeds, pumpkin seeds, sunflower seeds, leafy vegetables, and walnuts.

Saturated Fats

The fats we don't want to eat are the "saturated fats". These come from milk, cheese, meat, palm oil, coconut oil, and some seafood. Saturated fats raise your LDL (bad) cholesterol, and you want to avoid them as much as possible.

Trans Fats

These are cheap fats made for deep frying junk food like fries, donuts, and chicken in fast food restaurants. Trans fats are also used in packaged junk food like pastries, chips, and cookies. Read your labels! When you see trans fat, put the package down. Trans fats are in the "never eat" category.

Because we are concentrating on simple, natural foods, our list of best foods for healthy fats includes; eggs, nuts, avocados, olive oils, and limited amounts of fatty fish. We should aim for about 20% of our daily calories to come from fats. With a 1500 calorie diet, that means about 300 calories should come from good fats.

You must also keep in mind that many other foods have smaller amounts of fats. This has to be understood when planning what you eat for the day. Later on, we will get more specific about exactly what to eat. For now, it's enough to understand that you need all these basic building blocks in your diet, and they can all be obtained with simple, natural foods.

Minerals and Vitamins

In addition to the basic proteins, carbohydrates, and fats, we also need trace amounts of a long list of minerals and vitamins. The minerals we need are calcium, potassium, sodium, magnesium, phosphorus, and many others. The vitamins we need are vitamin D, vitamin E, vitamin A, and vitamin K, or the fat-soluble vitamins, and folate (folic acid), vitamin B12, biotin, vitamin B6, niacin, thiamine, riboflavin, pantothenic acid, and vitamin C. What a stroke of luck that by simply eating a *plant based diet* of fruits, vegetables, nuts and seeds, and some animal protein, you will automatically get all these minerals and vitamins in sufficient quantity.

Since changing my relationship with food to eat only whole, natural foods, I no longer bother with daily vitamin and mineral tablets.But if you are nervous about this subject, by all means take good qu ality daily vitamin and minerals separately. If you want to consider it as insurance, or if you don't trust the basic wholesomeness of the foods you will be eating, taking vitamins will not hurt anything but your wallet. Rest assured, you will get all the vitamins and minerals you require from your fresh, whole food diet. **Note:** *If you have a doctor' recommendation to add nutrition supplements, please do follow their directions.* I am not here to override your doctor's orders!

Once again, most of us can just trust Mother Nature. One of the most beautiful aspects of returning to whole, natural foods is that without much calculation, apart from basic portion control, you can trust that you are getting everything you need for optimum health. This is never possible with commercial diets, or even the more sophisticated "doctor diets." Before there were calorimeters, computers and scales, mankind was eating naturally by intuition, and doing perfectly fine. It was only the introduction of manufactured foods, chemical foods, junk foods, and faux foods that necessitated the precision calculation of each meal, or each processed food, in order to determine the nutritional content. The modern nutrition label found now on every packaged food was mandated for just this reason. In the age of processed foods, with so many artificial ingredients, and so many unrestrained and unrestricted advertising claims, no one knew what nutritional value, if any, was in the package.

Example: suppose you picked up a bag of unlabeled potato chips, thinking it is just fried potato slices. If these had been fried in very cheap palm oil, you would be getting a very heavy dose of unhealthy trans fats and saturated fats along with your simple potato.

The trans fat content would cancel out any healthy benefit of the natural potato—a very bad deal. The requirement for a label, spelling out all the nutritional elements of the product, allows you to see what potentially bad ingredients were used. That's certainly a help. But, we have a better, simpler and more powerful idea: Stay away from manufactured food all together, and you won't even need a nutrition label. You can think of that nutrition label as a legally mandated attempt to make food manufacturers more honest about the nutritional claims they make. Now pick up an apple or a banana, and please notice that *no nutrition label is required.*

Here's What I Ate Today

Here's a list of foods I eat on a typical day: Tomatoes, apples, an egg, 4 ounces of chicken, a handful of grapes, a banana, 1/2 potato, 1 teaspoon of peanut butter, 6 ounces of natural prune juice, a small whipped cream and strawberry dessert, and two dill pickles. Not in that order! All natural, all fresh and delicious. I had no need to calculate anything about the day's food, because I have been eating this way for a long time, and I can trust the contents. Some days are heavier on fruit, some on vegetables, but none are very heavy on meat, and at least half the days are free of meat.

Almost all of what I eat each day are "single ingredient foods" (SIFs). That means, the naked food by itself, not contained in some complicated recipe or prepared meal. I don't prepare meals. By "meals" I mean combining many ingredients through a recipe like Chicken Cacciatore, or Beef Bourguignon. That kind of meal preparation will invariably lead to overeating because the binding ingredients, mostly sauces, will have high quantities of fats and oils raising the caloric content. And, it's hard to serve the proper portions of complicated meals like that. It will also be spicy, that may contribute to digestive stress.

Eating SIFs is the best way to keep food unadulterated, natural, tasty and easy to digest. Use cooking only when it is required for meats, potatoes, beans, and steaming vegetables. There's always room for a couple exceptions. And, a few that are worthwhile are soups and stews. If you use all fresh ingredients, and avoid unnecessary salt and spices, home made soup is a great meal. Vegetable beef soup without the usual grains and rice, but with plenty of fresh vegetables, and just a tiny pinch of salt, is a perfectly good way to consume a little protein along with the vegetables. Be very selective about the broth you buy to make the soup. Salt content can be very high in some popular brands. Find the one with the lowest salt content. Another acceptable meal is cooking beans into a chili or bean soup. **WARNING! BEANS MUST BE COOKED!** Do not eat raw beans. Some varieties, like kidney beans, contain strong toxins that will make you very ill if eaten raw. Once more, don't be tempted to use too much spice, it defeats the purposes here. I will often make 6 quarts at a time of a rich vegetable beef soup with all fresh ingredients. This can be lunch for two for over a week and takes less than an hour to make.

Isn't this going to become very boring? Everyone assumes boring food is a bad thing—until they actually make the change and get a few weeks of the benefits under their belt. Is it boring to put the same brand of gas in your car every week? Is a stationary bike boring? Most exercise is boring, isn't it? I've used a treadmill in the past, and nothing was as boring as that. I imagine stationary bikes are also boring too. Since leaving the treadmill, I am now walking a circuit around my neighborhood each morning, and that is boring too after many trips day after day. But boring doesn't mean bad. Boring just means common, repetitive, routine and consistent. It is the consistency that brings the health benefits to food as fuel. There are no big surprises to your system—no "gut bombs.Is breathing clean air boring? Drinking fresh, clean water? It's only your over-active mind that was trying for so many years to make food exciting and adventurous that thinks eating healthy food is boring.

Let's just say eating right—eating for nutrition—is boring in the same way that breathing or drinking clean water is boring. Every single morning you wake up, your trillion cells, muscles and brain have the same nutritional demands they had the day before. They need the same proteins, carbohydrates, fats and minerals on Monday morning as on Friday morning. Are you going to make the task of nutrition easy, or make it harder for the sake of adding excitement? Does your system have to wade through piles of garbage to find the nutrients? Are you going to try to fool your cells with a gut full of beer and pizza? Mountains of donuts and cheese balls? Are you going to consume hundreds of useless chemical additives that your body must eliminate in order to find the nutrients? Would that be more exciting? How can good health be boring?

Food as fuel is the means to stop hurting yourself, stop fooling yourself about the purpose of food, and reverse the process for once and for all. Your stomach is not a garbage dump. *Food as fuel* is putting the highest grade gasoline in your tank, consistently, every single day, without harmful additives. It's no more boring than exercise or breathing. Get your excitement from the other things you will do when you have a healthy, trim body, and you can move around painlessly with ease. That's the promise I make to all who can find the desire to change. To all who can see the illogical behavior of trading your long term health for a few exciting moments with pizzas and cheeseburgers. Our bodies have mechanisms to protect the cells from poisons. Primarily, these are the liver and kidney functions. They remove harmful chemicals from the blood stream. As effective as they are, we don't want to perpetually overtax them on purpose. And yet, that's exactly what we do when we eat for excitement and adventure instead of good nutrition.

And, maybe it's not even as boring as I have made it sound already. After all, you get to eat pretty much all you want of some very delicious foods. Today's modern grocery stores are brimming with wonderful fresh foods all year long. Nothing prevents us from eating well and restoring our good health. Nothing that is, aside from a billion dollar advertising onslaught from the packaged food industry.

QUICK REVIEW

❊   Nature provides all the vitamins and minerals the body needs without any need for manufacturing and processing.

❊   Our bodies need water, protein, carbohydrates, fats and minerals for proper nutrition and all of this requirement can be found in fresh, whole, natural, single ingredient foods (SIFs).

❊   Cooking fancy recipes is not required to eat for nutrition.

❊   A large variety of fresh whole foods are available all year in the grocery store.

❊   Eating fresh is boring in the same way as breathing clean air, or drinking pure water.

❊   Processed food sends your liver and kidneys into overdrive trying to protect your body from toxins and foreign chemicals.

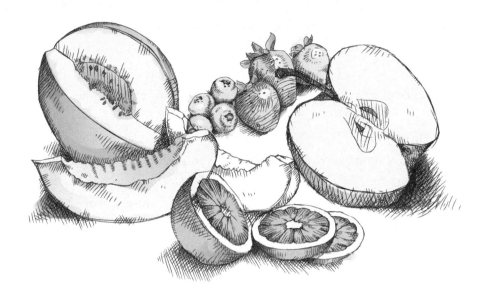

CHAPTER 6

How We Can All Get Fit and Thin

"Fit" and "unfit" are the terms I like to use for comparing our new body to our old body. Ironically, the commercial food culture is always presenting fit people in the promotion of food that is all but guaranteed to make you unfit. Their commercials tempt you with being fit, present you with only fit models, and then feed you in a way that assures you will remain unfit, and overweight. In this way, they maintain a high level of frustration, and a very high level of participation in their business of selling you ever more processed food. They intend for the population to yo-yo from diet to excess and back to diet again in a never ending cycle. But no matter where you are in that cycle, you are always buying more processed food. On the upswing you are buying exotic food experiences to entertain yourself, and on the downswing you are buying expensive diet foods, faux foods and chemical concoctions from the diet industry. What I am asserting in this book is that we can all be fit easily, with no yo-yoing up and down, no heartbreak, no pain, no torture, no will power, no surgery, no pills, no kidding—starting tomorrow!

Elitism

"You can never be too rich or too thin."—Wallis Simpson, Duchess of Windsor.

I don't subscribe to elitism at all. One's size, weight or medical condition, should never be a reason for such social discrimination and snobbishness. But, when it comes to your health, the evidence is overwhelming and convincing: *A lower BMI, barring rare disease, is going to lead to a longer healthier life.*

I am fully understanding of the social stigma in some cultures of being overweight. What really matters for us in this moment however, is the health aspect of our bodies. And on this, we know the logical, scientific answer: *It's statistically more advantageous to be thin and fit.* It reduces your odds of being burdened with a whole host of unpleasant diseases and conditions. It may extend your life by 10 or more quality years. There's no sensible reason for any human being to want to be burdened with disease and disability.

It's an all to common belief that not everyone can be fit. That some people are cursed with a special kind of slow metabolism, special DNA, unusual body type, or large bone structure, that dooms them to a life of being unfit, and overweight. There is another myth that some people can hardly eat any food at all, and still grow heavier each day. This is impossible, and has no basis in science.

It's like proposing perpetual motion or anti-gravity machines. Putting aside the rare disease, we become overweight because we eat too much of the wrong food too often.

While recent science is hinting that genetics play a role in becoming overweight, these genetic markers do not make it possible for you to put on weight without eating the necessary calories. The genetic role is that it causes some people to consistently overeat. It doesn't defeat the scientific principles that excess weight is the result of consuming too many calories.

It's important now to acknowledge the operation of science, because it is that very same science that will save us from the burden of being unfit, if only we will accept its basic principles. If you remain a believer in magic, you may as well put this book down, and go back to your "overeating then diet", roller coaster life. If you believe in magic, nothing but magic can ever help you, and I have no magic to offer. But, if you can accept the few simple science principles here, you can be as fit as the next person, and enjoy all the benefits of good health that it will bring. Magic or science? It is a simple choice.

Assuming you have accepted science over magic, you can easily understand why you have to get out from under the spell of the food culture. You are going to recognize that Asian fusion, or French cuisine, or Cajun cooking, has absolutely nothing to do with science or nutrition, and everything to do with eating for adventure, pleasure and excitement—a completely subjective experience.

Belief in the science of nutrition means that no matter what your weight condition is right now—no matter how much extra weight you are carrying—you can and will be thin and fit if you make the simple mental and physical commitment to food as fuel. If you are 200 pounds overweight, a few days from now you will be 199 pounds overweight. And in a few months you will be only 175 pounds overweight. Yes, it will take a while before you weigh 140 pounds again, as you did in your youth, but trust the truth of science that eventually you will be fit once more, and you will have the ability to stay that way in perfect harmony with your internal nature. Everyone can be fit and thin again.

Trust the Science

When you throw a golf ball and a bowling ball off the roof together, they will both hit the ground at the same time. It doesn't matter that one is 150 times heavier than the other. The scientific *Law of Gravity* predicts they will hit the ground together, and they do. Many people doubt this. It doesn't seem to make sense, and many people try their own experiments to disprove it. But in the end, they all see that the *Law of Gravity* is faithful, even for bowling balls and golf balls. In this same way, we can trust the *Law of Thermodynamics,* from which we derive this simple axiom: **calories consumed minus calories burned determines whether we gain or lose weight.**

If you eat 2000 calories today, and only burn 1500 calories, the excess 500 calories will go towards building excess fat. If you are overweight, you have fat pads over the muscles and organs of your body. Those fat pads were created by eating more calories than you can burn off each day, not by having bad genes, or because you have big bones, or because you have an unusual metabolism.

The fat is not created out of thin air, or by any magical process. The fat pads covering your organs and muscles are created by eating more calories than you burn, day after day, after day for many years.

A pound of fat is equal to 3,500 calories. If you consume 500 calories per day more than you burn off, in just seven days you will add one new pound of fat to your body (7 x 500 = 3500 calories). But it works equally well in reverse. If you consume 500 calories less than you burn, in seven days you will eliminate one pound of fat. This is all due to the physical *Law of Thermodynamics.* You can't create something out of nothing. Extra fat occurs from the food you eat and nowhere else. Let's all own the science, and agree that there is are no magical processes happening in our body. Accepting this simple scientific principle leads us immediately onto a path where we can have automatic success! Remember this: Just as there was no magic that created the fat, there is also no magic required to get rid of it! The logic works in both directions. This is why diets are totally unnecessary, and not useful. They are temporary patches to a permanent problem. This is also why there is no need of any special supplements or pills or formulas or drinks. That's all marketing propaganda. It's all designed by the food industry to keep you mystified about nutrition and weight loss. They try to make you accept the absurd premise that you need a special herb, or vitamin, or chemical potion in order to lose weight. That's not science, it's quackery. Actually, much of it is worse than quackery, it is fraudulent. It is preying on emotions of vulnerable people, desperate to regain control of their body.

Exercise

While we are at this point of accepting the science and logic of thermodynamics, let's talk about exercise. Our bodies all need exercise. We must move in order to maintain our health. The body is not a static plant or bio-blob. It has arms and legs and muscle systems designed to move, to carry, to bend, to lift, to walk and run. Without exercising these systems, we will die. So, at a minimum, we must agree that we have to keep moving as a part of our fitness and weight loss program. But we don't all have to become athletes. We don't even need to become joggers, or weightlifters, or bicyclists, or even swimmers. Just old fashioned *walking* is good enough. In fact, almost all medical experts would agree that walking is the very best exercise. We can all walk, unless we have a condition or disease that prohibits it, or we are just too large for our legs to carry us. In the first case of disability, we need to find alternate exercise, and only a physical therapist can prescribe what is best in each of those cases. If you are in that category, find one, and get some professional recommendations. You must find some suitable exercise. In the second case, of just being too large, we will move toward using walking as our basic exercise, even if it is only 10 feet at a time when you begin.

What we don't need to do is use exercise for weight loss. Here's why: exercise makes you hungry. And for casual exercisers, who are not athletes, too much exercise often leads to simply more overeating. I've seen this many times, and I bet you have too: A person rides a stationary bike for 30 minutes, and then makes a salad for lunch, topped off with a cup of nuts, croutons, some fruit, and then 500 calories worth of salad dressing oil! They falsely believe this is OK because they have exercised! But, the math will not work.

Riding that bike vigorously for 30 minutes will burn around 320 calories. That huge salad drenched in oil and high calorie toppings might easily be 500 calories. That's 180 more calories than were burned by the exercise! Walking casually only burns about 200 calories per hour. You can not walk your way to weight loss. It doesn't mean we shouldn't exercise. We want to use exercise to maintain our mobility muscles and improve our fitness. For weight loss, we are going to eat less, and eat the proper foods. We are going to start with the right diet, and then use exercise to improve our strength and mobility. This will be a far more successful path than trying to exercise off the fat. It can be summarize like this:

"Eat like a bird. Eat mostly plants. Move as much as possible."

Adopt these three simple principles and you will not need to buy any exercise machines, join any gyms, attempt to maintain impossible exercise regimes. Losing weight by exercise is a very difficult proposition. Not everyone is cut out for vigorous exercise, and many people don't even enjoy it. It would be awful if anyone was scared away from becoming thin and fit just because they thought too much exercise was involved. Some people are athletic by nature, and some are not. So, vigorous exercise is always an optional addition to this program if you are by nature an athletic person. But, you do not have to exercise to become thin. If you are able to ride bikes, row canoes and jog, great! Do those things because you love to do them, and have the body to do them, and would be doing them whether or not you had changed your eating habits. But, if you have two bad knees, a hip replacement, and are 100 pounds overweight, you do not have to commit to those extreme exercises to become fit and thin again. Let's instead focus on doing what we were made to do—walking. Once you are in the *food for fuel* mode, you will automatically become more energetic. Believe me, it just happens. Follow your own internal energy as it grows naturally, day by day.

Keeping Track of Weight Loss

Weigh yourself every single day without fail, and write it down on a weight loss log. Why is this necessary? First, because even small success is a motivator. Second, because you need to learn by example exactly how the Law of Thermodynamics works. I can tell you that, *calories in and calories out* is the only important fact you need to know, but like the gravity experiment of throwing balls off the roof, people learn better by seeing their own results. Unlike commercial diets, when you are on the *food for fuel* program your weight will go straight down, with no rebounds or bounce-backs. Every day you will weigh less than the day before. Maybe only a tenth of a pound or two per day, but it will go constantly straight down. There is only one complication to this, and that is the effects of water.

The Ins and Outs of Water

The human body is about 60% water. Your blood is 90% water. Your brain is mostly water, and even your bones are 20% water. That means in a 200 pound person, there is 120 pounds, or 17 gallons of water! Water is constantly flowing in and out of our body. Water leaves the body in our breath, through our kidneys as urine, through our skin as perspiration, and through our intestines and bowels.

We are constantly losing water that must be replaced throughout the day. Water only enters the body through the food, or by directly drinking water. We have a very hard time managing water exactly. We are never in perfect water balance. Our average content may be

17 gallons of water, but the actual amount is constantly changing depending on our exercise, our environment and our intakes.

There are medical conditions and their related drugs, like high blood pressure medications, that influence our water system. On average, we exchange (lose and gain) about 2.5 quarts of water per day. But, we don't make any practice out of exactly measuring our water intakes, and water losses. On a particular day you might take in 3 quarts of water and eliminate 2 quarts. On another day it might be reversed, with more water going out than coming in. For this reason, your weight, as measured on the scale, will include both your fat loss, and your water imbalance. It means that you will have lost fat, but because of a simple water imbalance for that day, the scale reads higher than the day before. The bigger you are, the bigger the water imbalance may be. So, when I say that you will be losing weight every day, I mean you should be *losing fat content every day,* but because of the imbalances possible in water, it might not always show up on the scale every day. By weighing yourself every day, you will be able to average out these imbalances, and see how they work. If you make a habit of weighing yourself at the same time every day, you will find the number has more consistency. To get the most consistent numbers, choose the very beginning of the day—before you have even had coffee or breakfast.

Waste Management

This is a subject that has to come up sooner or later in any discussion of nutrition and fitness. It's important in several ways for our *food as fuel* program. Of course, what we mean is the elimination of all body waste through the bowels. People caught in the food culture, eating large amounts of processed foods, often have great difficulty maintaining any semblance of regularity. Many people go days between bowel movements, and that is not what we want for optimum health. There is no end to the solutions offered by the food and drug industry, including special foods, over the counter drugs, and special herbal preparations. This is just more proof that eating such foods creates digestive difficulty.

We have no interest in these chemical laxatives, and do not recommend their use in this program. There is an easy natural remedy available, and that is our clear preference. Food takes on average a little over 12 hours to move through the digestive system. This is especially true of whole, natural, single ingredient foods that make up the bulk of our program. The simple mechanics dictate that all of the waste from any meal should be eliminated 12 to 24 hours after eating. Dense foods, with little dietary fiber, like cheese, meat, cookies, chips, and fried foods are a frequent contributor to constipation. Eating foods in their natural raw state is the easiest way to prevent it. When you eat light, eat fresh and eat natural whole foods, you will be amazed how easily and efficiently these pass through your digestive system. The objective for everyone should be to completely empty the bowels every single day. Start every day new, with an empty, ready to work, digestive system.

The foods you will be eating are high in dietary fiber already. But, if your system needs a small booster to get started on this daily routine, drink a 6 oz. glass of *regular prune juice* first thing each morning. Do not buy diet or "light" juice, that will contain chemical sweeteners, and do not buy it without pulp. Just buy traditional, regular prune juice, and add this to your morning routine. Prune juice is an entirely natural operator that contains *dihydrophenylisatin*, a natural laxative that creates bowel contractions. It also contains *sorbitol*, and other natural sugars, that bring water into the intestines to soften stools. While chemical laxatives are never recommended for daily use, prune juice is absolutely acceptable and desirable due to the natural cleansing action. While eating in this program, there is no concern regarding the 130 or so calories in your 6 oz. glass of prune juice. The major benefits of prune juice far outweigh the small caloric penalty. Just consider it to be part of your daily fruit intake.

QUICK REVIEW

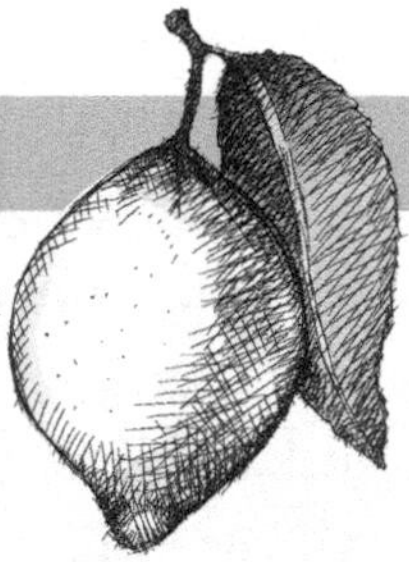

- Barring rare disease everyone can become fit and thin—that means a BMI of 20.
- Weight loss is pure science. *The Law of Thermodynamics* tells us that losing weight simply requires us to consume fewer calories than we burn off each day.
- We can not exercise our way to weight loss. We use exercise to increase mobility, and keep our muscle systems working well.
- In the *food for fuel* program, you will lose weight (fat) every day!
- During your weight loss phase, weigh yourself everyday, and record it.
- Try to increase your water intake as much as possible.
- Waste management is important! Use all natural prune juice daily for optimal results.

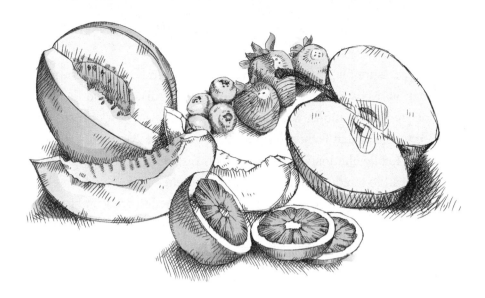

CHAPTER 7

The Importance of Good Health in Your Retirement Years

The link between obesity and high blood pressure is well established. Excess weight and obesity is the cause of 26% and 28% of high blood pressure in men and women respectively. An increase of fatty tissue throughout the body increases the vascular resistance to the flow of blood, and this raises the blood pressure. Having a BMI over 25 puts one at risk of developing high blood pressure. Also, "belly fat" or extra fat throughout the trunk, is an additional risk factor. This is indicated by a waist over 40" in men, and over 35" in women. *Over 60 million people in the United States are now being treated for high blood pressure.*

IMPORTANT: Always follow your doctor's recommendations for medications!

What is important to know is that losing weight is often a cure for high blood pressure. Even just a 10% weight loss can reduce blood pressure by 5 points. But, we don't want to shoot for a simple reduction, we want to completely eliminate the disease, and the associated medications, whenever possible. And the best chance of accomplishing that is by getting down to a BMI of 20. Even if that doesn't totally eliminate your high blood pressure, it will almost certainly lead to a reduction in the required medications to adequately control your high blood pressure. The steps needed are very simple:

✻ Eat fresh fruits, vegetables and small amounts of meat until your BMI is 20—that's our *food for fuel* program.
✻ Reduce alcohol consumption.
✻ Reduce sodium intake.
✻ Increase exercise.

Those are the four steps needed to help beat high blood pressure, and none of them are impossible for anyone.

The most unfortunate aspects of overeating are most pronounced on retirees. They have the hardest time losing weight because they are less active than most working people, and have more free time to overeat. Most retirees are on fixed incomes, and may be relying entirely on Medicare for their health insurance. Medicare doesn't cover everything, and adding unnecessary health problems caused by obesity can create a significant financial burden. As we get into the 60s, 70s and 80s, we are generally getting less exercise, and all too often we are eating more to fill the spare time. That's eating for entertainment. Anyone who has tried dieting after age 60 knows that it is much harder to lose weight than it was in your 20s or 30s. A look around you will reveal a precarious situation with more and more older people being disabled in old age just by being obese. They need canes, walkers, and even electric wheelchairs to get around. Reduced mobility further limits exercise. For many retired seniors, life is obesity, medications, endless doctor visits, compounding health problems, and severely limited mobility. That is depressing, and depression is often soothed by even more overeating. This does not have to be your life. Most of those problems are all the result of overeating bad foods, and all of that can be reversed today. It takes nothing more than developing your new understanding about the purpose of food.

There's nothing you can do about your genes whether good or bad. We can't change that today. But there's plenty you can do about the rest of your situation. With some care and attention to the basics you can stop making things worse because of your own choices. It's never too late to see the error and reverse course. You can begin today, and no matter how seriously obese you are now, you will be on the road to recovery tomorrow, and feel better within weeks. Within a year you will be a fountain of health and wellness. Eventually, you can get all the way back to that BMI of 20—a fit and thin person who is not burdened by medications, and who has the mobility and energy to enjoy your retirement years to the fullest. It almost sounds too good to be true, and yet it is scientifically true.

It doesn't appear that the medical community today is doing enough to reverse the course of their patients who are overweight and overeating. Many doctors offhandedly advise their patients to "lose some weight", but it would be a rare case where they provide the tools, knowledge, and monitoring to accomplish this goal. It's well beyond the doctor's role to monitor your diet on a daily basis. It's even well passed the average doctor's ability to recommend the right food for optimal nutrition. Of the 10 or 11 years of education a doctor receives, there may be as little as a few hours studying nutrition (almost half the medical schools in American provide no nutrition education). The Big Pharma companies are spending billions of dollars annually to advertise their latest drugs for all the common conditions of old age, and it's hard to see that they have any motivation to return customers to good health and fitness. Like the food industry, their core goal is always the same—always increase annual sales. They are quite happy to continue providing more expensive medications for hypertension, high cholesterol, and diabetes. All of that can largely be controlled by individual choices about food. To be blunt, the more diabetes and heart disease there is in the USA, the higher their profits will become.

If you are 65 years old now, you have already lived a life full of every food experience imaginable. How much more food pleasure do you really need? How many more prime ribs and triple chocolate cakes do you need to have completed that experience? Is it possible you can say, "been there, done that", and move on to a new phase of life designed to maximize your health? It's a choice you can easily make right now. As the elder in your extended family, you can also be a role model for your children and your grandchildren by establishing proper relationship to food. If you are still young, and have years to go before retirement, now is the chance to prevent all the problems we have been talking about. Any time is a good time to realign your relationship to food, and greatly enhance your fitness and well-being.

QUICK REVIEW

* The most common and preventable diseases of old age are diabetes and high blood pressure. Both can be cured through changes in diet and exercise.

* Very few doctors are qualified to instruct you on proper nutrition, as most have received no useful training in nutrition.

* The food and pharmaceutical industries have no incentive to improve your health. In the first case because eating less hurts their profits, and in the second case their profits are based on selling profitable treatments for disease.

* How much more exotic food experience do you need in life? Now, is always the best time to permanently change your relationship with food.

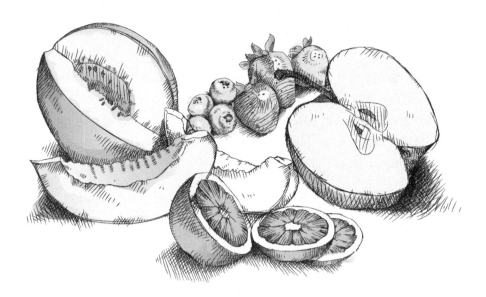

CHAPTER 8

Food for Fuel—What to Eat?

Now that you have committed to break up with the food culture, what exactly is it that you are going to eat for the rest of your life? In earlier chapters we described this as fresh fruits, vegetables, nuts, seeds and a small amount of meat. Now, we can get more specific.

First, let's review what we are never going to eat. Let's call this category "bad foods" to be perfectly clear about our intentions.

Bad Foods

Burgers, pizza, hot dogs, French fries, tacos, fried foods, chips, pretzels, and pork rinds

This junk is simply not healthy for anyone to eat. These fast foods pale in comparison to the healthy foods you could be eating. In an emergency you could get a fast food burger, ditch the bun and sauces, and just eat the burger patty, but that should be rare. Fast foods are the bargain basement of the food culture you are trying to avoid. It's just as easy to find a grocery store on that busy intersection as finding a burger joint.

Restaurant meals

Invariably these contain too large a portion, and lots of additives we don't want to eat. Restaurant food will also be served with breads, pastas and other grain products we do not want to eat. They will be over sweetened, over spiced, and over salted. When the meal arrives it is an unknown entity. Sure, it might taste good, that's the facet they control for your benefit. But, the ingredients can be extremely unhealthy. And, having paid for it, people are psychologically pre-disposed against waste, and will eat it all, regardless of portion size. Restaurants are temples of the food culture.

A popular restaurant meal of Italian food was recently analyzed to contain: 1,450 calories, 3,800 mg of sodium and 33 grams of saturated fat. Add to that a beginning salad, smothered in dressing, and you will have another 200 calories and 700mg of sodium.

That's about 3 days worth of sodium intake and a day's worth of calories in one meal! This is not unusual, it is typical.

Plan on just giving this up, except on the rarest occasion for special celebrations, where the social content is important to you and others. Then, just eat the small portions of meat and vegetables served, and skip the sauces, breads, and desserts.

Bread, pasta, cakes, crackers, cookies, pies, pancakes, waffles, muffins, bagels, pastries

If it has wheat, don't eat. After two weeks of being off these foods, you won't miss them at all. Remember, the problem with modern wheat grain is that is flips our hunger switch in the brain to ON, and causes us to want to eat beyond our satiation. Wheat is the super-charger of overeating.

Packaged commercial foods, breakfast cereal, canned soup, macaroni and cheese, frozen dinners, frozen pizza, snacks, candy

Don't buy prepared and packaged commercial foods. If it comes in a box or a can, don't buy it. The exception to packaged foods is fresh frozen vegetables, plain beans, and some meats and poultry. "Naked" frozen vegetables, those not smothered in sauces, are just as good as their fresh equivalents. They are only frozen for convenience, and can be considered as good as fresh.

Faux foods

This is my terminology for those dreadful concoctions brewed up by food scientists to imitate the "sin" foods you really want, by mixing nasty brews of taste and texture chemicals with no nutritional value. These Franken-foods are made and sold by commercial diet companies. They are sold as "low calorie" or "no/low fat" versions of sin foods, that would normally be on our bad foods list anyway. Making chocolate cake out of soy beans and flavor chemicals is nothing but a crutch—a substitute for what you really want— chocolate cake. Even though it can be argued that a faux cookie has less calories than a real cookie, it keeps you buried knee deep in the concept that food is for entertainment, pleasure and fun. That is not where we want to be. The longer you play with faux food, the worse your odds are of sustaining the weight loss. Eventually, your will power will crack, and you will want the real cookie, the real Danish, the real brownie. It's inevitable. And, once that starts, you are headed for failure. It is much better to train your tastes to want fresh fruits and vegetables, not faux foods.

Sugary drinks, diet soda

Many fruit juices now have added sugar that makes them every bit as bad as soda. Cranberry juices are loaded with high fructose corn syrup to make a tart, astringent, and not very tasty fruit, taste sweet enough to be enjoyed by millions. You however, should avoid it like the plague. Consuming sugar in drinks is the fastest way to add hundreds of useless calories to your diet.

Diet soda is no nutrition bargain. This is almost as bad as regular sugary soda. There are many potential hazards with the chemicals in diet soda. This is just not a good thing to consume because the long term effects of artificial sweeteners is under constant scrutiny. The preliminary study results do not look good. One of the emerging ideas in these studies is that artificial sweeteners dull your sense of taste for natural sugars found in fruits. This is because artificial sweeteners are hundreds, and in some cases thousands, of times sweeter than natural sugar. After repeatedly exposing your palette to these chemical demons, you will lose your taste and appreciation for the natural sweetness found in whole foods. These need to entirely disappear from your diet. Drink tea, water or juice before going down this artificial sweetener path.

Sugary Yogurt

Although plain yogurt is a healthy food, most brands of yogurt now have a lot of added sugar. This added sugar makes this kind of yogurt fall into the bad category in our program. Plain yogurt contains around 12 grams of natural sugars for 6 ounces. But the sugary yogurt, with fruits and added sugars, can be as high as 30 grams for the same 6 ounces. Worse yet, would be the *artificially sweetened* yogurts. If you don't like plain yogurt, forget it and take yogurt off your list.

The Good Food

The best foods are all those with just one ingredient—the naked food itself. Carrots and strawberries and apples and string beans are all *single ingredient foods* (SIFs). They stand on their own, and can be eaten as is, where is, with no preparation. Although light cooking can help with some of the very hard vegetables, it's not cooking in the sense of a recipe with ingredients. You don't need to add more ingredients, more spices, more flavors, more sauces, you just need to heat it or steam it to soften it. Many of the harder vegetables will be much more digestible after heating them.

Special note: other than green beans and string beans, do not eat beans or potatoes raw! Although potatoes are a good source of carbohydrates, they will not release their nutrients in the raw state. Not to mention they taste terrible. When raw, they will pass directly from the stomach into the intestines, and then begin to ferment. This will create very uncomfortable gas. The potato is not toxic per se, but not pleasant to eat raw.

The SIFs you should be eating are:

Carrots, peas, squash, beans, lettuce, spinach, celery, green beans, kale, broccoli, tomatoes, cucumber, asparagus, bell peppers, onions, cauliflower, cabbage, Brussels sprouts, zucchini, rutabaga, parsnip, rhubarb, radish, artichokes, beets, apples, pears, peppers, peaches, bananas, apricots, plums, berries, mangoes, watermelons, grapes, oranges, pineapples, grapefruits, tangerines, tangelos, cherries, kiwis, pomegranates, lemons, limes, plucots, Asian pears, plums, nuts, seeds. And, every other fresh whole food at your grocer!

These fruit and vegetable SIFs should make up the great bulk of your meals. I never use the phrase any more, "all you can eat", but you can eat a lot of these foods, and remain well inside the safe zone of daily calorie consumption to lose weight. The worst that could happen is that by eating too much fruit, you would consume too many calories for the day. Remember—a calorie is a calorie when it comes to weight loss. A calorie from a carrot is no different than a calorie from a chocolate brownie. But, with SIFs you won't be consuming chemicals, additives, spices, and preservatives, so if you are going to over eat, do it with fruits and vegetables. But, let's not consider overeating. We want to consider healthy amounts of these foods that will satisfy, while being highly nutritious fuel for the body. An excellent way to make vegetables into a delicious meal is to drizzle lemon juice over them in place of salad dressings, butter or oil.

More Good Food—Boutique Packaged Foods

There are some small boutique companies making unadulterated packaged food. You find these in the health food stores, and smaller specialty grocery stores. Check the label. Stay clear of added sugars, artificial sweeteners of any kind, and too many preservatives.

There is inevitably going to be a preservative in order to have some shelf life, but stay clear of long lists of chemicals and preservatives. And, for previous reasons, stay clear of wheat and pasta.

A good example of these boutique packaged foods are the many brands of frozen soy burgers, veggie burgers, and tofu products in general. There are several brands that are acceptable for regular consumption, and some others that would be suitable for occasional consumption. Because it is prepackaged, you have to be ever-vigilant regarding the ingredient labels.

More Good Food—Meats and Proteins

We must have proteins to survive, and animal proteins are the most complete. We must have what nutritionists call "complete proteins" to make the essential amino acids for survival. So, we are going to eat a little bit of meat, poultry, and fish to get these complete animal proteins into our fuel mixture.

Our target for daily total protein is 56g for men, and 46g for women. Don't forget, that protein is also in many of the other SIFs we will be eating, not just the meats. It would be a great misunderstanding to think you need "56g of meat protein" every day. Every food you eat will have some amount of protein. The meat, poultry and fish is added to the diet to be sure you get some of the "complete proteins" only found in meat, poultry and fish. Here are some examples of protein from meat, fish and poultry:

* 4 ounces of chicken is 36g of protein
* 4 ounces of beef is 28g of protein
* 4 ounces of salmon is 28g of protein
* 4 ounces of pork is 36g of protein
* 4 ounces of lobster is 20g of protein

As a general rule, a little bit of meat goes a long way. Let's be sure we know what a 4 ounce serving of chicken, salmon, or beef looks like. It's about the size of a deck of playing cards. By no means is it the whole half breast you generally see in the package. If you prefer beef, get the leaner cuts, and try to avoid the fatty ground chuck, although once in a while, that won't hurt you. You don't need to avoid all fats, you just need to consume them in moderation.

In addition to animal protein, let's also not forget that spinach, kale and broccoli are 45% protein. Other high protein foods include cauliflower, mushrooms, green peppers, nuts, figs, avocado, and eggs. What this means is that you don't need to eat a 4 ounce piece of chicken or beef every day to get your protein. If you are eating plenty of the high protein SIFs, you can reduce the amount of meat for any given day. Once you are eating these high nutrition foods, you will find that nutrition is almost automatic. That's the wonder of this food as fuel philosophy—it is naturally nutritious without a lot of work. You don't have to be a nutritional scientist. You only have to eat the foods on the list, and nature will take care of the rest. This is the reason I am not getting deep into the details of fats and oils, and other technical nutrition subjects, but rather recommending you read "Nutrition for Dummies," if you want to study that in detail. When most of your food comes from SIFs, and modest animal protein, you don't have to have a calculator, or a book full of charts and tables to eat optimally. It happens automatically!

More Good Food—Nuts and Seeds

These are a good source of protein, fiber, unsaturated fats, and other important minerals. They are anti-oxidants, and they fight inflammation. Walnuts, almonds, cashews, pecans, Brazil nuts and macadamia nuts are all good for you. These are foods you should always have on hand, and make them a small part of your daily routine. Don't eat a pound of nuts tomorrow. Actually, don't ever eat a pound of nuts! But a handful of nuts, 1 or 2 ounces a day, are absolutely an important part of your nutrition. You will discover that in most stores it is hard to find unsalted nuts and seeds. Keep looking, they are usually well hidden to favor the heavily salted "snack style nuts". You do not want to eat salted, or even lightly salted, nuts and seeds. Buy unsalted only, and eat in moderation, because they are very high in calories.

More Good Food—Eggs

Eggs have gotten a bad rap over the years as a contributor to high cholesterol. And, when lots of eggs are eaten with a poor diet, already filled with trans fats and saturated fats, they can be a contributor to high cholesterol. But in our diet, that is rich in fruits and vegetables, and ridiculously low in trans fats and saturated fats, eggs make an excellent source of protein, and should be no problem for most people. An exception to this would be those with severe diabetes. If that's you, limit your eggs to a few per week, or follow your doctor's direction.

More Good Food—Kefir

Kefir is fermented milk with a tart taste. It is made by adding cultured yeast and lactic acid (kefir grains) to milk. It is high in nutrients and has the special bonus of natural probiotics, an important aid to good "gut health". Kefir contains protein, calcium, Vitamin B12, Riboflavin, magnesium and phosphorus, and some Vitamin D, along with the bioactive compounds. In fact, kefir is a much more powerful bioactive than yogurt, offering over 30 strains of probiotic bacteria. A 6 ounce serving of milk kefir will contain 100 calories, 6 grams of carbohydrates and 5 grams of fat, depending on which milk is used to make the kefir.

Conditionally Good Food—Milk; cheese; soy, almond and rice plant-based drinks

Everything in this category is conditioned upon two general principles: 1. Don't consume any of these that are adulterated with chemical preservatives, or added sugars; 2. Don't consume a lot of your calories from this category.

For our purposes "milk" describes a product of animal lactation. Cow's milk, goat's milk and sheep's milk being the common varieties in western culture. Soy, almond, and rice beverages are also often branded as milk, but they are really combinations of plants, oils, water, and sometimes sweeteners, and artificial flavors. We call those plant-based drinks not milk.

Milk, and all these plant-based drink substitutes, is complicated enough for a whole book. Therefore, the first simplification, is to say that adults don't need to consume a lot of milk. But if you do like milk, it's best to avoid whole milk, which is high in saturated fats and calories. A bad choice. If you like milk in small amounts for cereal, or as a beverage, drink 2%, 1% or skim varieties. Milk is high in protein, calcium and vitamin D. But also high in saturated fat and calories. Avoid drinking whole milk.

Cheese should be considered "concentrated milk" for our purposes. Everything said about milk goes double or triple for cheese.

Yes, this is a natural food for the most part, and it is high in the same nutrients as milk, but with more concentrated calories! One ounce of cheddar cheese contains 24 grams of protein—we like that—but it also has a whopping 400 calories! This is a very calorie-dense food, so the important advice is to be cautious about serving size. Like milk, cheese is also available in reduced fat versions.

But when the fat is removed, so is most of the satisfaction. Enjoy, but tread lightly! This should not be the basis of many of your calories throughout the day.

Almond drink is made from water and ground almonds. It is low in calories and saturated fats, but also low in protein, whereas almond nuts are high in protein! Almond drink is a good source of vitamins A and D, and of course since it is not an animal product is lactose free. Keep in mind this product is primarily *water,* with a small amount of almond, and very often many additives. Read your label very carefully! This is conditionally a good food. But, if you see any added sugars, put this down and run. Almonds are great, and should be a part of your diet. Almond drink is an adulteration of fresh almonds, that enhances the profitability of almond growing by adding water, but has absolutely no advantage over the raw almond nuts. I don't see the point of this unless you really, really, love the taste as a beverage.

Soy milk offer the best nutrition of the plant-based drinks. Made from the soy bean plant, it is a good source of protein, vitamins A, D, B12, and potassium. It is cholesterol free, low in saturated fats, and has zero lactose. It has almost as much protein as milk, but the calories are comparable to skim milk. The down side is that some people have digestion problems with soy, and too much consumption has been shown to create some medical problems with fertility and sperm count. We would not recommend drinking that much of any of these plant-based drinks. In moderation, this can be a good substitute for milk. Watch out for any unwanted additives, like chemical flavoring, added sugar, or artificial sweeteners.

Rice drink is milled rice and water. It is very benign from an allergy point of view and might be suitable for those with nut or lactose allergies. Rice drink is high in carbohydrates and low in protein. That's not a combination we desire. So, this product should be considered only in small amounts, or for special reasons. Best advice is to the rice and drink a glass of water.

Food for Fuel—A Typical Day of Eating

What exactly might this way of eating look like on a typical day? I can offer some examples for me, but everyone will develop unique preferences, and eventually structure the meals to suit themselves. The wonderful thing is, there are no rules once you stay within the bounds of the natural, whole foods and avoid all the bad foods. Sure, the professional nutritionist will say you must eat ALL the varieties of vegetables, for example. But, we really don't need to be that perfect. If you love broccoli and hate spinach, that's OK—eat lots of broccoli. I absolutely guarantee that will be better for you than the frozen pizzas and bread you were eating. I happen to love peas, and on most days of the week, I am perfectly happy to eat a package of frozen peas with a teaspoon of butter on them for lunch!

That's it! Lunch is that simple, and that nutritious. Compare that to eating a submarine sandwich! Experiment and be creative. Try all the foods, and stick with the ones you like best.

Breakfast

1 scrambled egg and 1 (all natural and organic Aidells brand) chicken and apple sausage = 260 calories, and 25g of protein. Or, 1/2 cup traditional oatmeal with 1 sliced banana, and 1/4 cup of half-and-half = 310 calories, and 6 grams of protein.

Lunch

2 Roma tomatoes, 6 oz. serving of peas, or green beans with 1 tablespoon of salad dressing, and 1 apple = 320 calories.

Dinner

4 oz. serving of baked chicken breast, Brussels sprouts, fruit, apples, nuts = 600 calories, and 28g of protein.

Snacks

Fruits and nuts = 200 calories, and 6 grams of protein.

That comes to a total of about 1400 calories, and 40 to 60 grams of protein for the day. There is so much variety to choose from that no one should be bored. However, I prefer to eat the same things frequently, and I am not bored by that routine. I am not looking for a deep adventure or wild experience from my food, just 100% healthy nutrition. That's the essential meaning of *food for fuel*. Even so, what could be better than fresh, whole food for deliciousness?

I happen to love consistency, and I can easily eat the same things day after day. For me, it makes the *food for fuel* idea incredibly simple and predictable. But, I need to be aware that I don't eat past my hunger. In other words, like everyone else, I could easily fall into a phase of unconscious overeating if I lose my awareness of what I am doing: "Yum! These strawberries are soooo good, I will eat the whole container!" That's something to pay attention to, and recognize it when it happens. This doesn't mean I am starving or perpetually hungry. I am not. This way of eating isn't based on starvation. But having spent the first 65 years of life in the overeating food culture, there is always a reflexive tendency to eat from boredom, or to eat for the pure pleasure of eating—eating for fun. This tendency diminishes very rapidly once you are in the *food for fuel* lifestyle, but it will probably never totally disappear for modern westerners. We are just too well trained in the food culture, where every occasion is an occasion for eating. The bombardment of junk food advertising and promotion will never go away.

When you begin the program eat lots of vegetables. Make *that* your over indulgence in the beginning. Vegetables can be very filling, and yet will not wreak havoc on your blood sugar, or your weight. They are low in calories, and have a low glycemic index. A large bowl of broccoli, for example, will be very filling, but very healthy. You can't say that about cookies or chips.

In the overeating food culture, we have all expanded our stomachs, and it takes a lot to be satisfied. As you begin this new way of eating, just be mindful of your eating and try to gradually reduce the quantity over time. Your stomach will shrink to match your intake, and as you move forward you will begin to feel full and satisfied with less food. This is a natural process, and you don't need a surgical intervention to make this happen. People who insist on having surgical interventions to make their stomach smaller are really saying they want to remain in the food culture, but have some other power or mechanism forcing them to eat less. In other words, they want their cake, and to eat it too. That is the exact opposite approach that we want to adopt. We want to first get out of the food culture that is causing us to overeat, and then adjust our eating and food selection to be healthy. We don't need an outside force or intervention to have success. Breaking up with the food culture takes care of that.

As you go through the first week, be very aware of the portions you are eating. Try to reduce the portions gradually without feeling that you are starving. Although we definitely have the goal of eating less, the plan is not based on extreme denial, especially in the first few weeks. The food we want to cut out is the food that is being consumed just for entertainment, or being consumed out of boredom.

Gradually, you will be reducing your intake and shrinking your stomach, and losing weight. This is why it is crucial to weigh yourself every single day, and write it down. If you are not losing a pound or two the first week, you are probably still overeating. Try backing off a little at one meal. For many people breakfast and lunch are the easiest meals to reduce. Dinner is much harder. So, pick a meal, and then for the next week consciously reduce the quantity of what you are eating for that meal. Again, track your weight daily. You should now be losing a pound or two each week. Maybe even more in the beginning.

It's important to have some early success. We are all motivated by success. Once you find a combination that is allowing you to lose weight, and yet you are eating enough to be satisfied, stay with it. Once you have lost the first five pounds you will never turn back.

Notice that there has been very little discussion of *daily calorie counting* in this beginning phase. Commercial diets and doctor diets all begin with discussions about how many calories you can be allowed to consume. For women, it is usually suggested that around 2,000 calories a day is required for normal operation, and that for weight loss you will want to reduce that by 500 calories a day. Then they proceed to furnish manufactured meals of say, 500 calories each. You eat these meals three times a day, and it is presumed you will lose weight at the rate of 1 pound a week. e.g. 7 days x 500 calories a day = 3500 calories, or 1 pound. The problem is obvious to anyone: those meals are fixed, and your energy requirements might be changing from day to day. What do you eat if a particular meal, just wasn't enough? What do you eat if you just don't feel like eating the dreadful tasting *faux lasagna* today?

These manufactured meals are loaded with unnecessary ingredients, and plenty of preservatives and chemicals. Their flavors are entirely false because they are made up in test tubes full of chemical flavor enhancers. After a while, these false flavors become unappetizing, but that's all you have to eat. When that happens you will substitute on your own, and probably pick the wrong things to begin substituting. Many times you will choose breads, grains and snack foods because they tend to be most satisfying. But those wheat products can actually trigger more hunger! Next thing you know, you are overeating again.

This never happens on the *food as fuel* program. If on a particular day you need a little more, you just add a little more from the long list of delicious SIFs you have on hand. Only real flavors exist on our program, and you will not tire of them as you do with chemical foods. In fact, to the contrary, you will find that once you eliminate all the enhancers and chemicals, natural food in the natural state is delicious.

Your Fit, Thin Healthy Future—A Quick Summary

As we wrap this up, let's be absolutely sure we understand what has been presented here. Barring any rare diseases we might have, we are overweight because we are constantly overeating unhealthy, ultra-processed, commercially manufactured foods. Foods that do not occur in nature, but only in the minds of chemists and food engineers, who exist only to make food for profits. We've shown that that anyone can stop overeating if they switch to eating only fresh, natural whole foods, that we call food for fuel.

Being fit and thin is being healthy. By fit we mean a BMI of about 20. There's no doubt about that from any medical authority. Being thin and fit will greatly reduce the risks of common disorders like high blood pressure, diabetes and high cholesterol. Removing all your excess weight will very often allow you to effectively cure one or more of those disorders, and eliminate the medications that treat them. Of course, you will only change your medications on the advice of your doctor, but I can't imagine any doctor won't be amazed and delighted when you go from a BMI of 30 to a BMI of 20! Be prepared to amaze people.

There are many commercial and doctor diets available, but they just don't work over the long haul. Inevitably the weight comes back with a vengeance once the diet is over and you go back to your regular eating habits. That has been proven repeatedly by retrospective studies. The diet industry is relying on will power, and will power is not an infinite human resource. It eventually runs out.

What we propose is not a diet at all, it is a change in your understanding of the purpose of food. Food is not for fun, it is for fuel.

Keeping you overweight, keeping you constantly overeating, is the full-time job of the food culture. At the center of that food culture is the food and diet industry. They make ultra-processed, faux foods loaded with chemical preservatives, and flavor enhancers including the large amounts of sugar, salt and fat that are essential to the food industry. The role of every food company in the world is to grow their annual sales, and the only way they can do that is for you to grow in girth. When you eat more, they profit more. When they profit more, they advertise more. And, when you see more advertisements for food, you want to eat more. We are here now to put an end to that deadly cycle forever. We do this by *breaking up with the food culture* permanently, and realigning ourselves with food as fuel. It means getting out of the routines of restaurant eating, fast food eating, and so-called home cooking. It means we get rid of cookbooks, recipes, and highly prepared rich foods that sacrifice nutrition for a taste experience. In its place we choose whole, natural unprocessed foods that provide us with perfect natural nutrition. These single ingredient foods (SIFs) are all that is needed to find perfection in health. You do not need anything beyond these simple whole foods. They will provide you will every nutrient the body needs.

You also do not need any supplements, additives, pills or vitamins to have perfect health. Neither do we need any specially formulated diet foods and faux foods from the diet industry. None of that is desirable or necessary. The popular branded doctors' diets may be nutritionally correct, but they all require a lot of attention to specific calorie counting, and other strict rules. You don't need to do that either. Once you begin your food for fuel relationship with food, nature will take over, and all you need to do is follow some common sense. It really is that easy. Just trust Nature.

Big changes are hard to make. We have all grown up in the food culture and spent our entire life deeply involved with food for the wrong purpose. Just pay attention to those delectable food commercials that are exquisitely filmed in slow motion showing the butter sauce dripping off the lobster, and the sizzling steaks, and most of all, people laughing and having fun. These are really compelling story lines telling us food brings fun! Food brings friends! Food brings happiness! What's missing from those commercials?

Overweight and obese people. They always show people as thin as rails eating like hogs, and there's not an overweight person in sight. How much fun is it to be 100 pounds overweight? How much fun it is to be on 5 medications and spending all your disposable income on health care? How much fun is it to have to maneuver in an electric wheel chair because your knees have failed, and you can no longer walk? That's the part of the food culture story they never show. That's the reality of our overeating, food-for-fun, junk food culture. That's a reality you can say goodbye to forever, and start over right now!

Your friends and family will say this new *food for fuel* program is "too weird" or "too extreme." Be prepared. They may even makes jokes about you. Everyone in the food culture will try to lure you back in. They will have a million reasons why you should get back into what they call "eating normally." That's the way society works. Anything outside the normal behavior is considered too extreme. Give it a chance and see what they say in 6 months after you have lost 30 pounds, and are looking better than you have in many years! Give this program a chance for success, and you will be rewarded with a brand new life. There is absolutely no downside whatsoever to this program. Nothing you will be eating is bad for you. Nothing is negative. It is all 100% positive and healthy. Your new fit and thin self is out there waiting for you to say, *yes.*